Part 2 MRCOG: Single Best An

T0252192

Part 2 MRCOG: Single Best Answer Questions

Andrew Sizer
Shrewsbury and Telford Hospital NHS Trust, Shropshire, UK

Chandrika Balachandar
Walsall Healthcare NHS Trust, West Midlands, UK

Nibedan Biswas
Shrewsbury and Telford Hospital NHS Trust, Shropshire, UK

Richard Foon
Shrewsbury and Telford Hospital NHS Trust, Shropshire, UK

Anthony Griffiths
University Hospital of Wales, Glamorgan, UK

Sheena Hodgett
Shrewsbury and Telford Hospital NHS Trust, Shropshire, UK

Banchhita Sahu
Shrewsbury and Telford Hospital NHS Trust, Shropshire, UK

Martyn Underwood
Shrewsbury and Telford Hospital NHS Trust, Shropshire, UK

WILEY Blackwell

Library of Congress Cataloging-in-Publication Data

Names: Sizer, Andrew, author.
Title: Part 2 MRCOG : single best answer questions / Andrew Sizer, Chandrika Balachandar, Nibedan Biswas, Richard Foon, Anthony Griffiths, Sheena Hodgett, Banchhita Sahu, Martyn Underwood.
Other titles: Part two MRCOG
Description: Chichester, West Sussex ; Hoboken, NJ : John Wiley & Sons, Inc., 2016. | Includes bibliographical references and index.
Identifiers: LCCN 2015047746 | ISBN 9781119160618 (pbk.)
Subjects: | MESH: Obstetrics | Gynecology | Great Britain | Examination Questions
Classification: LCC RG111 | NLM WQ 18.2 | DDC 618.10076–dc23 LC record available at http://lccn.loc.gov/2015047746

Paperback ISBN: 9781119160618

A catalogue record for this book is available from the British Library.

Wiley also publishes its books in a variety of electronic formats. Some content that appears in print may not be available in electronic books.

Cover image: © selensergen/Gettyimages'

Set in 9/12pt, MeridienLTStd by SPi Global, Chennai, India.

1   2016

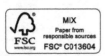

Contents

Notes on Authors

Andrew Sizer

Andrew Sizer completed specialist training in 2005 and was appointed as Consultant Obstetrician & Gynaecologist at Shrewsbury and Telford Hospital NHS Trust in 2007 and as Senior Lecturer at Keele University School of Medicine in 2008.

He is currently Clinical Director for Gynaecology and Lead Medical Appraiser for the Trust. He is the Chair of Intermediate training (ST3-5) at the West Midlands Deanery.

At the RCOG, he was a member of the Part 1 exam sub-committee from 2008 to 2011. At the end of this time he wrote 'SBAs for the Part 1 MRCOG' (RCOG Press) in conjunction with Neil Chapman.

From 2011 to 2014 he was Convenor of Part 1 revision courses. In 2014, he was appointed as Chair of the Part 1 exam sub-committee. He is an examiner for the Part 2 MRCOG.

Chandrika Balachandar

Chandrika Balachandar has been a Consultant Obstetrician and Gynaecologist at Walsall Healthcare NHS Trust since 1995. She has been Director of Postgraduate Medical Education for the Trust since 2010 and has established simulation training following training and certification as an instructor from the Center for Medical Simulation, Harvard, Cambridge MA. She is an examiner for Part 2 MRCOG since 2007 and coordinates the DRCOG examinations in Birmingham. She is a faculty member of the RCOG Part 2 revision courses, was a moderator for the RCOG Enhanced Revision Programme in 2013 and 2014 and member of the RCOG Assessment sub-committee from 2009 to 2012. From June 2015 she has taken on the role of Chair – Part 2 MRCOG Extended Matching Questions sub-committee. Mrs Balachandar is a generalist with special interests in High Risk Obstetrics, Colposcopy and Paediatric and Adolescent Gynaecology.

Nibedan Biswas

Nibedan Biswas completed his specialist training in Wessex Deanery in 2011 and worked as a locum Consultant at Poole hospital before joining Shrewsbury and Telford Hospital NHS Trust in 2012 as Consultant

Obstetrics and Gynaecology. He is the audit lead for the department and led the team that was successful in obtaining CNST level 3 status.

He is an undergraduate tutor for Keele University School of Medicine.

Richard Foon

Richard Foon started his professional career as a secondary school teacher before entering medical school.

He completed his training in Obstetrics and Gynaecology in 2012, which included 3 years of Subspecialty training in Urogynaecology in Bristol/Plymouth.

He has been a Consultant in Obstetrics and Gynaecology (with a special interest in Urogynaecology) at the Shrewsbury and Telford Hospital NHS Trust, since April 2012.

Currently, he is the Urogynaecology lead for the unit, the lead for Practical Obstetric Multi-Professional training and also the RCOG College Tutor.

Anthony Griffiths

Anthony Griffiths completed his specialist training in 2006 and was appointed as Consultant Obstetrician and Gynaecologist at the University Hospital of Wales the same year. He works closely with Cardiff University delivering postgraduate training for an MSc programme in ultrasound.

He holds postgraduate diplomas in both medical education and advanced endoscopy. He was awarded fellowship of the higher education academy in 2007.

Previously he served as an RCOG college tutor during 2006–2012 and is now Clinical Director for Obstetrics and Gynaecology. He is a preceptor for the ATSM in advanced laparoscopic surgery.

At the RCOG he was a member of the Part 1 examination subcommittee during 2011–2014. At that time he wrote an MRCOG Part 1 SBA resource. Since 2014 he has been convenor for the RCOG London Part 1 revision course. He also teaches on several international MRCOG courses.

Sheena Hodgett

Sheena Hodgett was appointed Consultant Obstetrician and Gynaecologist in 2000, and was initially at University Hospitals of Leicester prior to her appointment at Shrewsbury and Telford Hospital NHS Trust in 2009.

Her specialist areas of interest are intrapartum care and maternal and fetal medicine. She is the departmental lead for obstetric guidelines and for clinical research.

She is an examiner for Part 2 MRCOG having previously been a DRCOG examiner and undergraduate examiner at the University of Leicester. She has participated in MRCOG Part 2 courses in the United Kingdom and abroad.

Banchhita Sahu

Banchhita Sahu is a Consultant in Obstetrics and Gynaecology at the Shrewsbury and Telford Hospital NHS Trust. She completed specialist training in Obstetrics and Gynaecology in India and the United Kingdom.

She complemented her clinical training by working as a Clinical Research Fellow at University College London, a post with a substantial teaching and research commitment.

She has several first author publications in peer reviewed journals.

Her special interests include minimal access surgery, gynaecological oncology and simulation training in obstetrics and gynaecology.

Martyn Underwood

Martyn Underwood was appointed as Consultant Obstetrician and Gynaecologist to the Shrewsbury and Telford Hospital NHS Trust in 2014. He has interests in Ambulatory Gynaecology, Colposcopy and Minimal Invasive Surgery. He has taught on the RCOG Part 1 revision course for several years and also on the ACE Courses MRCOG Part 1 course in Birmingham. More recently, he has contributed to the Part 2 MRCOG course led by Andrew Sizer in Birmingham.

He has an interest in research in field of Gynaecology and Early Pregnancy and has recently contributed to several books in the field of Gynaecological Surgery.

Foreword

The RCOG's decision to add a Single Best Answer component to the Part 2 MRCOG examination was taken with the aim of making the examination more valid and relevant to clinical practice. I am therefore delighted to introduce this extremely useful and timely resource for candidates preparing for the new format of the examination.

The book's helpful layout mirrors that of the Curriculum to ensure full coverage of the relevant topics and their ease of reference by readers.

Candidates will find this book an invaluable aid to revision and examination practice when professional lives are increasingly busy and time is short. The authors have extensive experience of preparing candidates for MRCOG examinations and also of writing questions as members of the various College examination committees. As practising clinicians the authors are fully aware of the need to match theory to practice, and this book reflects the important role of the MRCOG in setting professional standards.

Dr Michael Murphy
Deputy Chief Executive
Royal College of Obstetricians and Gynaecologists

Preface

In 2014, cognizant of the introduction of single best answer (SBA) questions into the Part 2 MRCOG examination, a group of us, predominantly based in the West Midlands Deanery, decided to produce an SBA question resource.

Our aim was to produce questions mapped across the relevant modules of the curriculum and to use the following sources as our primary references:

RCOG Green top guidelines
NICE guidelines
Articles in 'The Obstetrician & Gynaecologist'

Between us we have produced 400 questions. The styles of the questions are different, but we envisage this will mimic the actual examination since many authors have contributed to the RCOG SBA question bank.

At the time of writing, very little was known about the actual style and content of SBA questions for the Part 2 MRCOG. We have used our experience and knowledge of medical education to develop questions that we feel are appropriate.

Knowledge accumulates, practice alters and guidelines change. We will be grateful for feedback.

We hope that candidates for the Part 2 MRCOG find this book helpful in their preparation for the examination.

For further examination practice for the Part 2 MRCOG, please visit www.andragog.co.uk

Acknowledgments

We would like to thank the following trainees for being our 'guinea pigs' in our initial attempts at question writing and for their useful feedback.

Dr Kiri Brown MRCOG

Dr Guy Calcott MRCOG

Dr Will Parry-Smith MRCOG

Dr Dorreh Charlesworth MRCOG

List of Abbreviations

BASHH	British Association for Sexual health and HIV
BHIVA	British HIV Association
CGA	RCOG Clinical Governance Advice
FSRH	Faculty of Sexual and Reproductive Healthcare
GTG	RCOG Green Top Guideline
NICE	National Institute for Health and Care Excellence
NICE CG	NICE Clinical Guideline
NICE IPG	NICE Interventional Procedure Guidance
RCOG	Royal College of Obstetricians & Gynaecologists
RCOG CA	RCOG Consent Advice
SIGN	Scottish Intercollegiate Guidelines Network
TOG	The Obstetrician and Gynaecologist

Introduction

Attainment of the membership to the Royal College of Obstetricians and Gynaecologists (MRCOG) is an essential component of specialist training in Obstetrics and Gynaecology in the United Kingdom. Possession of the MRCOG is also highly prized by specialists working in many countries worldwide.

In March 2015, there were some significant changes to the format of the written component of the Part 2 MRCOG examination, although there was no change in the syllabus.

Previously, the examination had consisted of short answer questions (SAQs), true-false (TF) questions and extended matching questions (EMQs). However, in order to keep abreast of modern thinking in medical assessment, the SAQs and TF questions were dropped in favour of single best answer questions (SBAs).

SBAs had already been introduced into the Part 1 MRCOG examination in 2012, so many candidates were familiar with them. From March 2015, the Part 1 exam consisted solely of SBAs.

Format of the Part 2 MRCOG Written Examination

The exam consists of two written papers with a short break (approximately 30 minutes) between them.

The two papers are identical in format and carry the same amount of marks.

Each paper consists of 50 SBAs and 50 EMQs, but the weighting between the two question types (reflecting the different format and time taken to answer) is different.

The SBA component is worth 40% of the marks and the EMQ component is 60%.

Each paper is of 3 hours duration, but in view of the weighting the RCOG recommends that candidates spend approximately 70 minutes

Part 2 MRCOG: Single Best Answer Questions, First Edition.
Andrew Sizer, Chandrika Balachandar, Nibedan Biswas, Richard Foon,
Anthony Griffiths, Sheena Hodgett, Banchhita Sahu and Martyn Underwood.
© 2016 John Wiley & Sons, Ltd. Published 2016 by John Wiley & Sons, Ltd.

on the SBA component and 110 minutes on the EMQ component. There are however, no buzzers or warning regarding this, so candidates are responsible for their own time management.

Traditionally, Paper 1 is mainly Obstetrics and Paper 2 mainly Gynaecology, but there is no guarantee that this is the case and theoretically, any type of question or subject could appear in either paper.

Why Have SBAs Been Introduced?

SBA questions have been used as a form of written assessment for decades in a variety of subjects at a variety of levels, but have found increasing use in undergraduate and postgraduate medical examinations over the past 15 years as well as in the General Medical Council (GMC) assessment of poorly performing doctors.

SBAs allow much wider coverage of the syllabus when compared to SAQs and questions can be mapped to the entire syllabus using a blueprinting grid.

Compared to TF questions, SBAs are considered to be a higher level form of assessment. When considering their assessment ability according to Millers pyramid, they can assess 'knows how' and 'knows' as opposed to 'knows' alone (see Figure 1).

An SBA question usually consists of an introductory stem, which in a clinical question could recount a clinical history or scenario. There is then a lead-in question that should ask a specific question. Following this, there will be five options, one of which is the correct, or best, answer.

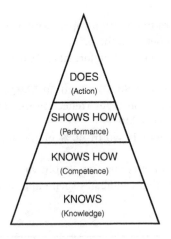

Figure 1. Millers Pyramid (see Miller, 1990)

There are therefore two variations of SBAs: single 'best' answer where one of the answer stems is clearly more appropriate or better than the rest, although the other answer stems are plausible, and the single 'correct' or single 'only' type of question where only one stem is correct and the remaining are incorrect.

Where SBAs are used for basic science questions in medical examinations the single 'correct' type of question tends to predominate, since the answers are generally very clear-cut. However, when SBAs are used to assess clinical knowledge, the single 'best' type of question predominates since clinical scenarios and their management tend to be more open to interpretation, or, indeed, there may be more than one type of management that is perfectly reasonable.

A good SBA question should pass the 'cover test', meaning that in a properly constructed question a good candidate should be able to cover the answer options and deduce the answer merely from the information in the stem and the lead-in question. In practice this can be difficult, and question writers often resort to a 'which of the following ... ' style of questioning. However, this is not a true SBA and is really a true-false question in the guise of an SBA.

Our advice would be always to apply the cover test. In other words, read the question with the five options covered. If you feel you know the answer and it appears in the list of options, your answer is almost certainly correct. A well-constructed question will have plausible 'distractors' that could make you doubt yourself. Therefore, it is best to try and answer the question without initially looking at all the options.

There are a number of potential flaws in SBA questions, which the well-prepared candidate could possibly use to their advantage. Many of these (with examples) are summarised in Hayes and McCrorie (2010). In addition to these, numerical questions will have a preponderance of answer 'C' being correct. This is because it is more common to spread the 'distractors' around the correct answer. However, the wily question writer can use this phenomenon to his advantage and place the correct numerical answer at either end of the spectrum.

We hope that our 400 questions give a broad coverage of the syllabus and that you will find the different styles of question writing useful. However, as Obstetrics & Gynaecology is such a vast subject, it is impossible to cover everything unless the questions run into several volumes.

We have not included questions in core modules 1, 2, 4 and 19 as we do not feel these subjects lend themselves to the SBA format and can be better assessed by other assessment tools. The number of questions in the included core modules represent what we consider to be an appropriate weighting.

We hope you find this book helpful as part of your exam preparation.

References

Hayes, K and McCrorie P (2010) The principles and best practice of question writing for postgraduate examinations. Best practice & research Clinical Obstetrics and Gynaecology, 24, 783–794.

Miller, GE (1990) The assessment of clinical skills/competence/performance. Academic Medicine, 65, S63–S67.

Questions

Questions

Module 3

IT, Governance and Research

1 If involved in a serious incident requiring investigation (SIRI), initial steps would involve completing an incident form, ensuring completion of notes accurately and participating in team debrief.
If a trainee is involved in an SIRI, what action should be taken as soon as possible?
A. Discuss with the medical defence organisation
B. Engage fully with the investigation
C. Meet with the educational supervisor to discuss the case
D. Write a formal statement
E. Write a reflection of the vent

2 In surrogacy arrangement, the commissioning couple need to obtain parental orders. Within what time frame after delivery must these be made?
A. 6 months
B. 12 months
C. 18 months
D. 24 months
E. 36 months

3 When managing a patient with surrogate pregnancy, who decides about the treatment required for any clinical situation that may affect the pregnancy?
A. The binding agreement
B. The commissioning father
C. The commissioning mother
D. The surrogate mother
E. The unborn child

Part 2 MRCOG: Single Best Answer Questions, First Edition.
Andrew Sizer, Chandrika Balachandar, Nibedan Biswas, Richard Foon,
Anthony Griffiths, Sheena Hodgett, Banchhita Sahu and Martyn Underwood.
© 2016 John Wiley & Sons, Ltd. Published 2016 by John Wiley & Sons, Ltd.

4 A primigravida at 24 weeks gestation has come to the antenatal clinic with a fear of childbirth and is asking for elective caesarean section as a mode of delivery.

What would be the recommended management?

A. Adequate exploration of the fears with counselling by trained personnel

B. Discharging the patient to midwife care with advise for vaginal delivery

C. Enlisting the patient for elective caesarean section

D. Referral to another obstetrician for second opinion

E. Referral to the supervisor of midwife

5 Women requesting caesarean section on maternal request might have posttraumatic stress disorder (PTSD) after previous childbirth. What is the incidence of PTSD after childbirth?

A. 0–1%

B. 6–7%

C. 12–13%

D. 24–25%

E. 36–37%

6 Among those receiving gynaecological treatment, what is the reported incidence of domestic violence in the United Kingdom?

A. 11%

B. 21%

C. 31%

D. 41%

E. 51%

7 When obtaining consent for a procedure, a doctor should take reasonable care in communicating with the patients, as their inability to recall from such discussion is often evident.

What percentage of the information that is discussed during the process of obtaining consent before surgery is retained at 6 months?

A. 10%

B. 20%

C. 30%

D. 40%

E. 50%

8 One of the main challenges faced by clinical trials is a lower than expected rate of recruitment.

What is the key to successful recruitment?

A. Collaboration and collective effort in multicentric trials

B. Do nothing, as clinical trials are not important

C. Provide incentives for participation in medical studies

D. Wait for colleagues to publish clinical trials

E. Withhold care to patients if they do not agree to participate in clinical trials

9 Improved outcomes are often observed in women participating in a clinical trial.

What is the reason behind this improved outcome, irrespective of study findings?

A. Positive change in the behaviour of clinicians and participants along with improved delivery of care

B. There is no difference in the outcome of care

C. Treatment is provided in a new hospital with latest technology

D. Treatment is provided in a tertiary hospital

E. Treatment is usually based on postal delivery of medication

10 On completing a consent form with a patient for a diagnostic laparoscopy, you mention that the chance of suffering a bowel injury is 'uncommon'.

How would you define 'uncommon' in this context in numerical terms?

A. 1/1–1/10

B. 1/10–1/100

C. 1/100–1/1000

D. 1/1000–1/10,000

E. <1/10,000

Module 5

Core Surgical Skills

11 A medical student asks you how to measure blood pressure.
What maximum pressure should you inflate the cuff to measure systolic blood pressure in pregnancy?
A. Always initially inflate to 200 mmHg then deflate
B. Patient's palpated diastolic blood pressure
C. Patient's palpated systolic blood pressure
D. Patients palpated systolic blood pressure + 20–30 mmHg
E. Patients palpated systolic blood pressure + 5 mmHg

12 A healthy 39-year-old woman with no significant past medical history attends a preoperative assessment clinic.
She is due to undergo a total abdominal hysterectomy for heavy menstrual bleeding following a local anaesthetic endometrial ablation that was unsuccessful.
She is fit and well.
What preoperative investigation is required?
A. Chest X-ray
B. Coagulation screen
C. Electrocardiogram
D. Full blood count
E. Renal function tests

13 On deciding where to place your secondary lateral ports at laparoscopy, care should be taken to avoid the inferior epigastric vessels.
Where can these be found?
A. ~2 cm from the midline
B. Lateral to the lateral umbilical ligaments
C. Lateral to the medial umbilical ligaments
D. Medial to the lateral umbilical ligaments
E. Medial to the medial umbilical ligaments

Part 2 MRCOG: Single Best Answer Questions, First Edition.
Andrew Sizer, Chandrika Balachandar, Nibedan Biswas, Richard Foon,
Anthony Griffiths, Sheena Hodgett, Banchhita Sahu and Martyn Underwood.
© 2016 John Wiley & Sons, Ltd. Published 2016 by John Wiley & Sons, Ltd.

14 Your hospital has recently had an increase in postoperative infections. As a result, you are formulating a new guideline that includes information on skin preparation and hair removal prior to surgery. What is the most appropriate method of hair removal prior to surgery?
  A. Electric clippers
  B. Electrolysis
  C. Laser
  D. Shaving
  E. Waxing

15 Following delivery, a woman is found to have a third degree tear and a trainee wishes to do the repair under supervision.
  Which two suture materials have equivalent efficacy when repairing the external anal sphincter?
  A. Polydiaxanone (PDS) and chromic catgut
  B. Polydiaxanone (PDS) and nylon (Prolene)
  C. Polydiaxanone (PDS) and Polyglactin (Vicryl)
  D. Polyglactin (Vicryl) and chromic catgut
  E. Polyglactin (Vicryl) and nylon (Prolene)

16 A 45-year-old woman is undergoing an abdominal hysterectomy for a history of heavy menstrual bleeding that has not responded to medical treatment. The patient has a past history of pelvic pain and the operation notes from a previous laparoscopy comments that the patient had 'pelvic adhesions'
  What is the most appropriate action in terms of protecting the ureter?
  A. Identify the ureter tracing it from the pelvic brim and mobilise the ureter by incising the peritoneum and sweeping the tissues laterally
  B. Mobilise the entire ureter with the aid of electrosurgery to reduce the blood loss
  C. Perform a preoperative MRI
  D. Perform a preoperative MRI and Intravenous urogram to assess the ureters
  E. Perform preoperative ureteric stenting

17 A 45-year-old asthmatic patient attends the gynaecology clinic with heavy menstrual bleeding and an ultrasound scan suggests the presence of an endometrial polyp.

The patient is booked for an outpatient hysteroscopy.

What analgesia should be prescribed at least 1 hour before the procedure?

A. Buprenorphine
B. Diclofenac
C. Ibuprofen
D. Paracetamol
E. Tramadol

18 What is the preferred distension medium for outpatient diagnostic hysteroscopy?

A. Carbon dioxide
B. Dextran
C. Glycine
D. Icodextrin
E. Normal saline

19 At what pressure should the pneumoperitoneum be maintained during the insertion of secondary ports for a laparoscopic procedure?

A. 5–10 mmHg
B. 12–15 mmHg
C. 20–25 mmHg
D. 30–35 mmHg
E. >35 mmHg

20 What is the background rate of venous thromboembolism in healthy non-pregnant non-contraceptive using women?

A. 0.5/10,000/year
B. 2/10,000/year
C. 5/10,000/year
D. 10/10,000/year
E. 20/10,000/year

Module 6

Postoperative Care

21 What proportion of patients having a surgical procedure will develop a surgical site infection?
   A. 5%
   B. 10%
   C. 15%
   D. 20%
   E. 25%

22 What is the most common source of microorganisms causing surgical site infection?
   A. Anaesthist
   B. Contaminated surgical equipment
   C. Patient
   D. Postoperative nursing staff
   E. Surgeon

23 A 54-year-old patient has had an insertion of a mid urethral retropubic tape and following the procedure there was a significant fall in the haemoglobin levels from 12.3 g/dl to 7.8 g/dl. Imaging investigations show the presence of retropubic hematoma. A decision is made to evacuate the hematoma. The most appropriate incision would be:
   A. Cherney incision
   B. Kustner incision
   C. Maylard incision
   D. Midline (median) incision
   E. Pfannenstiel incision

Part 2 MRCOG: Single Best Answer Questions, First Edition.
Andrew Sizer, Chandrika Balachandar, Nibedan Biswas, Richard Foon, Anthony Griffiths, Sheena Hodgett, Banchhita Sahu and Martyn Underwood.
© 2016 John Wiley & Sons, Ltd. Published 2016 by John Wiley & Sons, Ltd.

24 A postoperative patient who had a hysterectomy received morphine in recovery and then again in the gynaecology ward. Her respiratory rate is suppressed; she is drowsy and has pinpoint pupils.

What medication would you give to reverse this potential morphine overdose?

A. Atropine

B. Buprenorphine

C. Flumazenil

D. Naloxone

E. Pethidine

25 A patient who is frail, old and overweight has undergone a midline laparotomy and pelvic clearance for an endometrial cancer.

On postoperative day 4, the nursing staff notice that she has a pressure ulcer with full thickness skin loss, but the bone, tendon and muscle are not exposed.

What type of pressure ulcer grade is this?

A. Grade 1

B. Grade 2

C. Grade 3

D. Grade 4

E. Grade 5

26 A woman had an emergency caesarean section for a pathological CTG and pyrexia in labour. She was discharged on postoperative day 4 but re-admitted on day 6 with pyrexia, tachypnoea, tachycardia and hypotension. Haemoglobin is 105 g/l.

Septic shock is the main differential diagnosis.

Following the Sepsis 6 bundle, along with antibiotics and blood cultures, which other important blood test needs to be taken?

A. C-Reactive protein

B. Fibrinogen

C. Lactate

D. Urea and electrolytes

E. White Cell Count

27 A patient undergoes a challenging hysterectomy. A drain is left in the pelvis. You are called to review the patient eight hours later as the nurses have noted a high serous drain output and poor urinary output.

What finding would identify if the drain fluid is urine (suggestive of a bladder/ureteric injury) or normal peritoneal fluid?

A. Peritoneal creatinine > urine nitrogen

B. Peritoneal urea > urine urea

C. Serum creatinine > peritoneal creatinine

D. Serum nitrogen > drain fluid nitrogen levels

E. Urine nitrogen > peritoneal nitrogen

28 A patient has a ventouse delivery. Two days later she reports general malaise, fever and feeling unwell.

With sepsis, which is the first clinical sign to deteriorate, which can be detected through the use of early warning scores?

A. Altered consciousness

B. Hypotension

C. Hypoxia

D. Tachycardia

E. Tachypnoea

29 Oral fluids and food are often delayed following major gynaecological surgery.

Which gastrointestinal complication is improved by early postoperative feeding?

A. Abdominal distension

B. Incidence of diarrhoea

C. Need for nasogastric tube placement

D. Recovery of bowel function

E. Rectal bleeding

30 Following a difficult hysterectomy, a 65-year old woman has returned to the gynaecology ward. She had large amounts of morphine in the recovery area for pain relief and is also connected to a patient-controlled analgesia device.

The nurses note that she is drowsy and her respiratory rate is low. The anaesthetist decides to perform arterial blood gas sampling.

What disturbance of acid–base balance is this most likely to show?

A. Metabolic acidosis

B. Metabolic alkalosis

C. No disturbance

D. Respiratory acidosis

E. Respiratory alkalosis

Module 7

Surgical Procedures

31 Which type of ureteric injury is most commonly reported at laparoscopy?
A. Crush
B. Laceration
C. Ligation
D. Thermal
E. Transection

32 During laparoscopic pelvic surgery, which visceral structure is most likely to be damaged?
A. Aorta
B. Bladder
C. Ileum
D. Rectum
E. Ureter

33 Theoretically, what kind of injury related to laparoscopic entry should be reduced by the Hasson (open) technique, compared to a Veress needle entry?
A. Bladder injury
B. Bowel injury
C. Major vessel injury
D. Splenic injury
E. Ureteric injury

Part 2 MRCOG: Single Best Answer Questions, First Edition.
Andrew Sizer, Chandrika Balachandar, Nibedan Biswas, Richard Foon,
Anthony Griffiths, Sheena Hodgett, Banchhita Sahu and Martyn Underwood.
© 2016 John Wiley & Sons, Ltd. Published 2016 by John Wiley & Sons, Ltd.

34 An 18-year-old nulliparous girl presents as a gynaecological emergency with severe left-sided pelvic pain, tachycardia and vomiting. A pregnancy test is negative. An ultrasound scan is performed in the emergency department, which appears to demonstrate a left adnexal cyst.

In theatre, a laparoscopy is performed which shows an ovarian torsion that has twisted three times on its pedicle. The left tube and ovary appear purple and congested.

What is the most appropriate surgical management?

A. Convert to laparotomy and perform a left salpingo-oophorectomy

B. Laparoscopic left salpingo-oophorectomy

C. Untwist the tube and ovary and perform a laparoscopic ovarian cystectomy

D. Untwist the tube and ovary and perform a oophoropexy

E. Untwist the tube and ovary, drain the ovarian cyst and leave the tube and ovary in situ

35 A patient undergoes a laparoscopic cystectomy for a dermoid cyst and some spillage of the contents occurs into the peritoneal cavity. What will be the incidence of chemical peritonitis?

A. 5%

B. 15%

C. 25%

D. 35%

E. 45%

36 When comparing robotic-assisted surgery to conventional laparoscopic surgery for gynaecological procedures, what would be the major drawback?

A. Intraoperative complication rate

B. Length of hospital stay

C. Operative time

D. Postoperative complication rate

E. Safety and effectiveness in gynaecological cancer

37 A 19-year-old is undergoing a laparoscopy for pelvic pain. What is the estimated risk of death due to a patient undergoing a laparoscopy?

A. 1 in 100

B. 1 in 1000

C. 1 in 10,000

D. 1 in 100,000

E. 1 in 1,000,000

38 A 22-year-old is undergoing a laparoscopy for suspected endometriosis.

What is the estimated risk of bowel, bladder or blood vessel injury?

A. 1.2:10,000

B. 2.4:10,000

C. 1.2:1000

D. 2.4:1000

E. 4.8:1000

39 Consent is being obtained from a 24-year-old for a diagnostic laparoscopy and it is correctly documented that there is a risk of laparotomy if any injury to bowel, bladder or blood vessels were to occur during the procedure.

The patient wishes to know what proportion of cases would be converted to a laparotomy should an injury occur?

A. 17%

B. 31%

C. 48%

D. 67%

E. 92%

40 A healthy 54-year-old lady is due to attend the outpatient post-menopausal bleeding hysteroscopy clinic.

Which medication should she be advised to consider taking prior to her attendance at the clinic?

A. Benzodiazepines

B. non-steroidal anti-inflammatory agents (NSAIDs)

C. Opioids

D. Paracetamol

E. Prostaglandins

41 A 62-year-old is due to undergo a hysteroscopy due to a thickened endometrium detected as part of her investigations for postmenopausal bleeding.

Which medication should be used to 'prime' the cervix prior to the hysteroscopy?

A. Mifepristone

B. Misoprostol

C. No medication required

D. Non-steroidal anti-inflammatory

E. Vaginal oestrogen

42 A 43-year-old lady with a history of heavy menstrual bleeding and a scan suggesting a polyp is due to undergo an outpatient hysteroscopy.
Which distension medium is routinely recommended due to its improved quality of image and speed of the procedure?
A. Carbon dioxide
B. Gelofusin
C. Normal saline 0.9%
D. Purosol
E. 5% glucose

43 A 32 year old is due to undergo a laparoscopic operation for investigation and management of an ovarian cyst detected on scan.
What is the expected serious complication rate following a laparoscopy?
A. 1:500
B. 1:1000
C. 1:2500
D. 1:5000
E. 1:10,000

44 With respect to instrumentation of the uterus, which operation has the highest risk of perforation?
A. Division of intrauterine adhesions
B. Outpatient hysteroscopy
C. Postpartum suction evacuation for haemorrhage
D. Second generation endometrial ablation
E. Surgical termination of pregnancy

45 What is the most frequently encountered complication of suction evacuation of the uterus for first trimester miscarriage?
A. Haemorrhage
B. Pelvic infection
C. Perforation
D. Retained products of conception
E. Significant Cervical Injury

46 A 19-year-old woman is to undergo a laparoscopy for pelvic pain. How would you describe the correct technique for entry with the veress needle?
  A. Enter below the umbilicus horizontally and then pass the needle at 45° to the skin
  B. Enter below the umbilicus transverse plane and then pass the needle at 45° to the skin
  C. Enter below the umbilicus vertical to the skin
  D. Enter at the base of the umbilicus and pass the needle at ~60° to the skin
  E. Enter the base of the umbilicus vertical to the skin

47 What is the most common complication of the bottom up single-incision retropubic tape procedure?
  A. Bladder perforation
  B. De novo urinary urgency
  C. Retention
  D. Tape erosion
  E. Voiding dysfunction

48 You have attempted to perform a direct entry for your laparoscopy and opted to undertake a Palmer's point entry.
  Where would you find Palmers point?
  A. 1 cm below the left costal margin in the mid-clavicular line
  B. 1 cm below the right costal margin in the mid-clavicular line
  C. 3 cm below the left costal margin in the mid-axilla
  D. 3 cm below the left costal margin in the mid-clavicular line
  E. 3 cm inferior to the right intercostal margin

49 A laparoscopic hysterectomy has been completed and several port sizes have been used.
  When the port is in the midline, what size of port requires closure of the rectus sheath?
  A. <5 mm
  B. 5 mm
  C. 7 mm
  D. >10 mm
  E. All midline ports

50 A laparoscopy oophorectomy has been completed and the port sites are about to be closed.
What diameter of nonmidline port site required closure of the rectus sheath?
   A. No nonmidline port
   B. <5 mm
   C. 5 mm
   D. >7 mm
   E. All midline ports

51 A woman is due to undergo an outpatient hysteroscopy and is concerned about pain.
Which hysteroscope is associated with the least discomfort in the outpatient setting?
   A. All are the same
   B. Flexible Hysteroscope
   C. Rigid Hysteroscope 0°
   D. Rigid Hysteroscope 15°
   E. Rigid Hysteroscope 30°

52 A woman is due to undergo an outpatient hysteroscopic polypectomy using a bipolar resectoscope.
Which distension medium should be used?
   A. Glucose 5%
   B. Glycine
   C. Manitol
   D. Normal Saline
   E. Purisol

53 A woman is due to undergo a routine diagnostic laparoscopy.
According to RCOG data what is the expected incidence of bowel injury during a laparoscopy?
   A. <0.1/1000
   B. 0.36/1000
   C. 3.6/1000
   D. 3.6/10,000
   E. 3.6/100,000

54 A woman with a stage 3 uterine prolapse is considering a variety of surgical options.

She understands the potential benefits of a mesh repair but is concerned about the risk of mesh erosion.

What is the risk of mesh erosion for a patient undergoing a subtotal hysterectomy with sacrocolpopexy?

A. 4%

B. 7%

C. 14%

D. 18%

E. 24%

55 A woman had a total abdominal hysterectomy in the past using a lower transverse incision.

She has now developed a persistent ovarian cyst and is due to have a laparoscopic bilateral salpingo-oophorectomy.

What will be the incidence of adhesions in the region of the umbilicus in this scenario?

A. 11%

B. 17%

C. 23%

D. 31%

E. 45%

56 A morbidly obese woman is due to undergo a total laparoscopic hysterectomy for endometrial cancer.

What type of complication is more common compared to traditional open hysterectomy in this situation?

A. Bowel injury

B. Hernia

C. Infection

D. Urinary tract injury

E. Venous thrombosis

57 A woman has been offered a sacrocolpopexy for a vault prolapse. Her friend had a similar operation but developed stress incontinence following the procedure.

What is the incidence of de novo stress incontinence after a sacrocolpopexy?

A. 1–5%

B. 7–12%

C. 14–19%

D. 21–26%

E. 27–32%

58 A woman presents with a history of dysuria, postmicturition dribble and vaginal discharge.

On examination, a tender mass anteriorly inside the introitus is found. You suspect a urethral diverticulum.

What investigation would you use to diagnose the presence of a urethral diverticulum?

A. Urethroscopy using a 0° endoscope
B. Urethroscopy using a 12° endoscope
C. Urethroscopy using a 30° endoscope
D. Urethroscopy using a 70° endoscope
E. Urodynamics

59 A 45-year-old multiparous woman is due to have a hysterectomy for heavy menstrual bleeding. The patient is considering having a subtotal hysterectomy as she has had normal cervical smears history.

When comparing a subtotal hysterectomy to a total hysterectomy, which perioperative complication is reduced?

A. Bowel injury
B. Cyclical vaginal bleeding
C. Intraoperative blood loss
D. Pyrexia
E. Urinary retention

60 At the end of a total laparoscopic hysterectomy (in which the woman was placed in a steep Trendelenburg position) you observe that the woman's shoulder brace was placed too laterally.

What type of nerve injury may present in the postoperative period?

A. Femoral nerve injury
B. Lower brachial plexus injury
C. Radial nerve injury
D. Ulnar nerve injury
E. Upper brachial nerve injury

Module 8

Antenatal Care

61 A nulliparous woman with a dichorionic diamniotic twin preg-
nancy presents at 32 weeks gestation with severe pruritis and an
erythematous papular rash on her abdomen with periumbilical
sparing. The most likely diagnosis is:
A. Atopic eruption of pregnancy
B. Eczema
C. Obstetric cholestatsis
D. Pemphigoid gestationis
E. Polymorphic eruption of pregnancy

62 A woman presents at 34 weeks gestation with a sudden onset of
severe headache and altered consciousness following an episode
of vomiting and diarrhoea. What is the most appropriate imaging
technique?
A. Cerebral angiography
B. Computerised tomography (CT scan)
C. Magnetic resonance imaging (MRI scan)
D. Magnetic resonance venography (MRV scan)
E. Skull X-ray

63 A woman attends for a dating ultrasound scan at 12 weeks ges-
tation. Doppler ultrasound identifies tricuspid regurgitation and a
reversed A-wave in the ductus venosus (DV). She is at increased
risk of which condition?
A. Early onset fetal growth restriction (FGR)
B. Early onset pre-eclampsia
C. Fetal anaemia
D. Fetal aneuploidy
E. Late onset pre-eclampsia

Part 2 MRCOG: Single Best Answer Questions, First Edition.
Andrew Sizer, Chandrika Balachandar, Nibedan Biswas, Richard Foon,
Anthony Griffiths, Sheena Hodgett, Banchhita Sahu and Martyn Underwood.
© 2016 John Wiley & Sons, Ltd. Published 2016 by John Wiley & Sons, Ltd.

64 A woman is referred by the community midwife with suspected small for dates pregnancy at 33 weeks gestation. Ultrasound assessment confirms a small for gestation (SGA) fetus with reduced liquor volume and reversed end diastolic flow on umbilical artery (UA) Doppler. Cardiotocograph (CTG) is normal. What is the most appropriate management?
A. Antenatal steroids and delivery within 1 week
B. Elective delivery at 37 weeks gestation
C. Immediate delivery by caesarean section
D. Repeat Doppler ultrasound in 1 week
E. Repeat ultrasound growth assessment in 2 weeks

65 What proportion of pre-eclampsia can be predicted by risk assessment from maternal history alone in the first trimester of pregnancy?
A. 10–20%
B. 20–30%
C. 30–40%
D. 40–50%
E. 50–60%

66 When aspirin is used to reduce risk of pre-eclampsia in woman at high risk, at what gestation should it be commenced for maximum efficacy?
A. Before 12 weeks
B. Before 16 weeks
C. Before 20 weeks
D. Before 24 weeks
E. Before 28 weeks

67 When calcium supplementation is used to reduce the risk of pre-eclampsia in women at high risk, at what gestation should it be commenced?
A. 12 weeks
B. 16 weeks
C. 20 weeks
D. 24 weeks
E. 28 weeks

68 What proportion of pregnant women in the United Kingdom is estimated to take the recommended dose of periconceptual folic acid supplementation?
A. less than 5%
B. 5–10%
C. 10–20%
D. 20–50%
E. 50–70%

69 What is the incidence of red cell antibodies in pregnancy?
  A. 1 in 500
  B. 1 in 300
  C. 1 in 160
  D. 1 in 80
  E. 1 in 40

70 In the presence of anti-c red cell antibodies in pregnancy, which additional red cell antibody increases the risk of fetal anaemia?
  A. Anti-D
  B. Anti-e
  C. Anti-E
  D. Anti-Fy^a
  E. Anti-K

71 A woman attends the antenatal clinic following a scan at 36 weeks gestation in her fourth pregnancy, which identifies an anterior placenta previa. She has had three previous caesarean births. What is the risk of placenta accreta?
  A. 3%
  B. 11%
  C. 40%
  D. 61%
  E. 67%

72 What proportion of pregnant women in paid employment require time off work due to nausea and vomiting of pregnancy (NVP)?
  A. 10%
  B. 20%
  C. 30%
  D. 40%
  E. 50%

73 What is the incidence of acute appendicitis in pregnancy?
  A. 1 in 400 to 1 in 800
  B. 1 in 800 to 1 in 1500
  C. 1 in 1500 to 1 in 2000
  D. 1 in 2000 to 1 in 2500
  E. 1 in 3000

74 A 21-year-old woman is admitted at 22 weeks gestation in her first pregnancy with suspected appendicitis. She has a low grade pyrexia with a leucocytosis and a mildly elevated C reactive protein level. Abdominal ultrasound is inconclusive. What imaging technique is the most appropriate subsequent investigation?

  A. Abdominal X-ray
  B. Computed tomography (CT) scan of the abdomen
  C. Magnetic resonance imaging (MRI) scan of the abdomen
  D. Repeat abdominal ultrasound in 24 hours
  E. Transvaginal ultrasound scan of the pelvis

75 What is the risk of serious neonatal infection associated with prelabour rupture of membranes (PROM) at term?

  A. 0.5%
  B. 1%
  C. 1.5%
  D. 2%
  E. 2.5%

76 A women in her first trimester scores more than 3 in the 2-item Generalized Anxiety Disorder scale (GAD-2) used to identify anxiety disorders in pregnancy.

  What is the best plan of care?

  A. Further assess using the GAD-10 scale
  B. Further assess using the GAD-7 scale
  C. Reassure
  D. Repeat the GAD-2 scale in 4 weeks
  E. Repeat the GAD-2 scale in second trimester

77 Women suffer from various anxieties in pregnancy.

  What is tokophobia?

  A. Fear of baby dying in utero
  B. Fear of extreme pain
  C. Extreme fear of childbirth
  D. Fear of heights
  E. Fear of spiders

78 What vitamin should women be advised to be taken throughout pregnancy and also while breastfeeding?

  A. Folic acid
  B. Vitamin A
  C. Vitamin C
  D. Vitamin D
  E. Vitamin K

79 An 18-year-old woman books into the antenatal clinic at 12 weeks of gestation. She is fit and well but is noted to have an increased body mass index (BMI) but no other risk factors for diabetes.
What BMI and above should she be offered screening for diabetes?
A. 25
B. 30
C. 35
D. 38
E. 40

80 An anxious woman attends the antenatal clinic. She is planning an afternoon picnic and has a list of her favourite foods including UHT milk, cottage cheese sandwiches, vegetable pate, lambs kidneys and baked oily fish.
Which of these food products is not recommended in pregnancy due to the risk of listeriosis?
A. Cottage cheese
B. Lamb's kidneys
C. Oily fish
D. UHT milk
E. Vegetable pate

81 A woman is advised to avoid drinking all alcohol in pregnancy but she declines. She enjoys wine but no more than 250 ml per week. She is keen to understand the safe limits of alcohol intake.
What is acceptable with regard to alcohol intake during pregnancy?
A. 1–2 UK Units per week
B. 3–4 UK Units per week
C. 5–6 UK Units per week
D. 7–8 UK Units per week
E. 9–10 UK Units per week

82 A women presents with vaginal candidiasis at 23 week pregnancy. What treatment should you offer her?
A. One stat treatment of live yogurt
B. One stat treatment of topical imidazole
C. One week course of oral Ketoconazole
D. One week course of oral nystatin
E. One week course of topical imidazole

83 You have been asked to review a full blood test results of a woman at 28 weeks of gestation. At what threshold level of haemoglobin concentration would you define anaemia at this gestation?
   A. 90 g/l
   B. 95 g/l
   C. 100 g/l
   D. 105 g/l
   E. 110 g/l

84 A pregnant woman undergoes a routine anomaly ultrasound scan at 18 weeks of gestation. No ultrasound soft markers are present. At what nuchal translucency measurement is it recommended to refer the woman to fetal medicine services?
   A. 2 mm+
   B. 3 mm+
   C. 4 mm+
   D. 5 mm+
   E. 6 mm+

85 A woman is noted to have a low-lying placenta at her 20-week anomaly scan. At what gestational age should you arrange the next scan to assess placental localisation?
   A. 28 weeks
   B. 30 weeks
   C. 32 weeks
   D. 34 weeks
   E. 36 weeks

86 A woman declines an induction of labour at 42 weeks of gestation, the indication being 'post-dates'. What is the recommended for assessment of 'fetal wellbeing' in this situation?
   A. CTG three times a day
   B. CTG twice daily and weekly Doppler assessment of the umbilical arteries blood flow
   C. CTG twice weekly with an assessment of deepest vertical pool of liquor on ultrasound
   D. CTG weekly with Doppler of the umbilical arteries
   E. Weekly Doppler assessment of the umbilical arteries blood flow only

87 A woman at 36 weeks of gestation presents with an uncomplicated breech presentation and consents to undergo an external cephalic version (ECV) after consultation. Unfortunately, due to logistics, this service will not be available when she is 37 weeks.

What management is most appropriate?

A. Elective caesarean section at 37 weeks

B. Elective caesarean section at 38 weeks

C. ECV at 36 weeks

D. ECV at 38 weeks

E. Induction of labour 37 weeks to avoid potential cord prolapse

88 A pregnant woman at 34 weeks gestation is complaining of severe chronic sleep problem.

What would be the most appropriate pharmacological intervention?

A. Diazepam

B. Fluoxetine

C. Imipramine

D. Lithium

E. Promethazine

89 A woman undergoes a successful external cephalic version at 37 weeks gestation.

What is the chance of spontaneous reversion to breech?

A. <5%

B. 6–8%

C. 10–12%

D. 14–16%

E. 18–20%

90 Which tocolytic agent has been proven to increase the success of an ECV?

A. Glyceryl trinitrate (GTN) patch

B. Glyceryl trinitrate (GTN) sublingually

C. Magnesium sulphate infusion

D. Nifedipine

E. Terbutaline

91 A Gravida 3, Para 2 (both full term normal deliveries) is diagnosed with breech presentation at 35 + 1 weeks of gestation and is keen to have an external cephalic version.

At what gestation is external cephalic version recommended for this mother?

A. 35 weeks
B. 36 weeks
C. 37 weeks
D. 38 weeks
E. 39 weeks

92 A primigravida aged 26 is admitted with threatened preterm labour at 30 weeks and seeks counselling with regards to antenatal corticosteroids.

What are the three recognised fetal benefits associated with antenatal corticosteroid administration in the case of premature delivery?

A. Reduced respiratory distress syndrome, reduced incidence of hypoglycemia, reduced neonatal death rates
B. Reduced respiratory distress syndrome, reduced VII nerve damage, reduced incidence of hypoglycemia
C. Reduced respiratory distress syndrome, reduce incidence of pneumothorax formation, reduced retinal disease of prematurity
D. Reduced respiratory distress syndrome, reduced intraventricular haemorrhage reduced neonatal death rate
E. Reduced respiratory distress syndrome, reduced intraventricular haemorrhage reduced necrotising enterocolitis rates

93 A woman who had a previous second trimester miscarriage is currently undergoing a serial ultrasound assessment of cervical length. With what cervical ultrasound feature would cervical cerlage be recommended?

A. Cervical length less than 25 mm before 24 weeks of gestation
B. Cervical length less than 30 mm before 24 weeks of gestation
C. Cervical length less than 45 mm before 24 weeks of gestation
D. Funneling of the internal os and a cervical length less than 30 mm
E. Funneling of the internal os before 24 weeks of gestation

94 A woman at 32 weeks gestation is admitted with severe falciparum malaria. What is the pharmacological treatment of choice?
   A. Artesunate
   B. Chloroquine
   C. Primaquine
   D. Quinine
   E. Quinine and glucose infusion

95 A woman who is in the second trimester of pregnancy is planning to travel to an area endemic for chloroquine-resistant malaria. What would you recommend as the drug of choice for prophylaxis?
   A. Artusenate
   B. Chloroquine
   C. Mefloquine
   D. Nonpharmacological preventative agents
   E. Quinine

96 The velocimetry measurement of blood vessels can be used to improve perinatal outcomes in high-risk pregnancies. Which vessel is assessed?
   A. Middle cerebral artery
   B. Umbilical artery
   C. Umbilical vein
   D. Uterine artery
   E. Uterine vein

97 A gravida 2 Para 0 + 1 molar pregnancy is diagnosed with Rhesus isoimmunisation. Doppler assessment of which vessel is used to monitor fetal anaemia during pregnancy
   A. Middle cerebral artery
   B. Umbilical artery
   C. Umbilical vein
   D. Uterine artery
   E. Uterine vein

98 A woman presents at 26 + 5 weeks of gestation in her first pregnant with reduced fetal movements. What is the most appropriate initial investigation to carry out?
   A. Biophysical profile
   B. CTG
   C. Doppler auscultation
   D. Ultrasound biometry
   E. Uterine artery Doppler

99 Domestic violence during pregnancy increases the risk of maternal mortality.

What is the increase in homicide risk when there is domestic violence during pregnancy?

A. twofold

B. threefold

C. fourfold

D. fivefold

E. sixfold

100 A woman who is 28 weeks pregnant in her first pregnancy attends the antenatal clinic. She has no medical problems, but on routine questioning, she discloses domestic abuse. She insists that this information has not been disclosed to anyone else.

What is the first action that should be undertaken?

A. Contact the Police

B. Contact the Independent Domestic Violence Advocate (IDVA) for advice

C. Document the consultation fully in the hand-held record

D. Perform a safety assessment

E. Persuade the woman to leave her partner and seek refuge in a shelter

101 A course of antenatal corticosteroids is associated with a significant reduction in neonatal morbidity and mortality in women who are at risk of preterm birth.

What is the reduction in risk of intraventricular haemorrhage?

A. 5%

B. 12%

C. 26%

D. 46%

E. 68%

102 What proportion of twin pregnancies have monochorionic placentation?

A. 10%

B. 25%

C. 33%

D. 50%

E. 67%

103 What proportion of monchorionic twin pregnancies are compli-
cated by twin to twin transfusion syndrome (TTTS)?
A. 1–2%
B. 10–15%
C. 25–30%
D. 50–60%
E. 70–80%

104 A woman with a monchorionic diamniotic twin pregnancy at 25
weeks gestation is assessed at the regional fetal medicine service.
She is found to have severe TTTS (Quintero stage III).
What is the optimal treatment?
A. Amnioreduction
B. Fetoscopic laser ablation
C. Septostomy
D. Termination of the donor twin
E. Termination of the entire pregnancy

105 A 30-year-old primagravida with a BMI of 28 is seen in the ante-
natal clinic at 36 weeks gestation following referral from the com-
munity midwife with suspected 'large-for dates'.
An ultrasound scan is arranged, which confirms the fetus to be
large for gestational age.
An oral glucose tolerance test is arranged a few days later, which
is normal.
What is the correct management?
A. Elective caesarean section at 38 weeks
B. Elective caesarean section at 39 weeks
C. Induction of labour at 37 weeks
D. Induction of labour at 40 weeks
E. Induction of labour at 40 weeks + 10 days

106 In the United Kingdom, the perinatal mortality rate is approxi-
mately 7 per 1000 births.
What is the perinatal mortality rate in monoamniotic twin
pregnancies?
A. 10–30 per 1000
B. 30–70 per 1000
C. 100–300 per 1000
D. 300–700 per 1000
E. 700–900 per 1000

107 A healthy 35-year-old woman attends the antenatal clinic at 37 weeks gestation in her third pregnancy. She has had two previous caesarean sections for breech presentation, but the current pregnancy has a cephalic presentation and she would like to have a vaginal birth after caesarean (VBAC).

What would be the risk of uterine rupture if she labours with such a history?

A. 0.4–0.5%

B. 0.7–0.9%

C. 0.9–1.8%

D. 2.5–3.1%

E. 4.8–6.7%

108 A 41-year-old woman with a BMI of $36 \, kg/m^2$, but otherwise healthy, attends the antenatal clinic at 14 weeks gestation and is found to have a dichorionic diamniotic twin pregnancy.

What supplementation would you advise to reduce her risk of developing pre-eclampsia?

A. Aspirin 75 mg daily until 28 weeks

B. Aspirin 75 mg daily until term

C. Aspirin 150 mg daily until 34 weeks

D. Calcium 1 mg daily until 20 weeks

E. Calcium 10 mg daily until term

109 During pregnancy, how much calcium is accumulated by the fetus?

A. 1–2 g

B. 10–15 g

C. 25–30 g

D. 70–100 g

E. 150–200 g

110 A 26-year-old primagravida with a singleton pregnancy at 23 weeks gestation attends for an ultrasound scan following a small amount of vaginal bleeding.

It is noted that the cervical length is 21 mm.

What is the appropriate management?

A. Antenatal corticosteroids

B. Expectant management

C. Insertion of a McDonald suture

D. Insertion of a Shirodkar suture

E. Tocolytic therapy

111 Which protein is the most important biomarker for the detection of PPROM (Preterm Prelabour Rupture of Membranes)?
   A. Nitrazine
   B. Placental alkaline phosphatase
   C. Placental Alpha Microglobulin-1 (PAMG-1)
   D. Placental vasopressinase
   E. Pregnancy-associated plasma protein A

112 What is the usual method of diagnosing placental abruption?
   A. Clinical diagnosis
   B. D-dimer level
   C. Kleihauer test
   D. Transabdominal ultrasound
   E. Transvaginal ultrasound

113 A primigravida with a low-risk pregnancy is admitted at 30 weeks with an antepartum haemorrhage (APH). A diagnosis of placental abruption has been made. The bleeding settled with conservative management and she is discharged home.
   What is the most appropriate plan for her further antenatal care?
   A. Advise continued hospital stay
   B. Reassure and continue with midwife-led care and arrange for induction of labour at term + 10 days
   C. Reassure and continue with midwife-led care as the bleeding has settled
   D. Reclassify as 'high risk' and arrange consultant-led care
   E. Reclassify as 'high risk', arrange consultant-led care with serial ultrasound for fetal growth

114 A 35-year-old primigravida is seen in the antenatal clinic for booking. She had been diagnosed with breast cancer at the age of 32 and received adjuvant chemotherapy with doxorubicin following surgery.
   What is the most appropriate management?
   A. Advice termination of pregnancy
   B. Arrange echocardiography to detect risk of cardiomyopathy
   C. Arrange outpatient ECG and 24 hour cardiac monitoring to detect risk of cardiomyopathy
   D. Make a referral to the Oncologist
   E. Reassure and plan consultant led antenatal care

115 You receive a telephone call from a community midwife. A 22-year- old primigravida, currently 15 weeks pregnant, has developed chickenpox and the rash had developed 72 hours ago. The mother is very anxious and the midwife requests advice with regard to further management.

What would you advise?

A. To inform the mother about the risk of fetal varicella syndrome and advice termination of pregnancy once she overcomes the infective stage

B. To reassure the mother and a course of Aciclovir to be obtained from the General Practitioner

C. To reassure the mother and arrange for VZIG administration from the General Practitioner

D. To reassure the mother that the risk of spontaneous miscarriage is not increased and arrange referral to a fetal medicine specialist for further advice and a detailed ultrasound

E. To reassure the mother that the risk of spontaneous miscarriage is not increased and arrange referral to a fetal medicine specialist for amniocentesis to rule out Fetal Varicella Syndrome

116 A 22- year- old Sudanese Asylum seeker is seen for booking in the antenatal clinic at 12 weeks. She is a primigravida and an ultrasound scan revealed a singleton pregnancy appropriate for gestation. She has history of female genital mutilation (FGM) and examination reveals Type II FGM.

What would be the he most appropriate management?

A. Defibulation during first stage of labour

B. Defibulation during second stage of labour

C. Elective caesarean section at 38 weeks to avoid labour

D. Elective defibulation at 20 weeks

E. Episiotomy only for second stage

117 A gravida 2 Para 1 + 0 attends the antenatal clinic for booking at 14 weeks. Her previous pregnancy was an emergency caesarean section for abruption at 38 weeks. Dating scan confirms a live fetus with a low risk for Down's syndrome. Routine bloods indicate her to have blood group B Rh negative and the antibody titre performed 2 weeks prior to the appointment reveals the anti-D level to be 5 IU/ml.

With regards to hemolytic disease of the fetus and newborn (HDFN), what is the optimal management?

A. Arrange for her partner's blood group to be tested for his Rhesus status

B. Enquire if she received anti-D following the previous pregnancy and delivery

C. Make a referral for fetal medicine opinion due to risk of HDFN

D. Reassure the mother that the HDFN is unlikely at that level and advice repeat assessment at 28 weeks

E. Repeat the blood test in 2 weeks to assess the anti-D levels again

118 A primigravida complains of recurrent herpes at 32 weeks gestation. She has been treated with Aciclovir at 20 weeks for a primary episode of genital herpes. She would opt for caesarean section if Herpes lesions are detected at the onset of labour.

What would you advise?

A. Administer intravenous Aciclovir now and arrange elective caesarean at 39 weeks

B. Advice supportive treatment only for now and daily suppressive Acyclovir from 36 weeks

C. Advice supportive treatment only for now and intravenous therapy during labour

D. Reassure that the risk of neonatal herpes is very small and discharge back to midwife care

E. Repeat another course of oral Aciclovir and advice intravenous therapy during labour

119 A primigravida is seen for booking. She is 40 years and has conceived through IVF. Ultrasound scan has confirmed a twin pregnancy. Her BMI is 36 kg/m².

What treatment would you advise to reduce the risk of pre-eclampsia ?

A. Aspirin 75 mg daily
B. Folic acid 5 mg/day
C. Low molecular heparin 40 mg subcutaneously daily
D. Low salt diet
E. Vitamin C & E

120 A community midwife requests advice with regard to induction of labour for a woman who is currently 40 weeks gestation. She has had 2 previous vaginal deliveries at 38 and 39 weeks. The pregnancy has been uncomplicated.

What would you advise?

A. To arrange induction as soon as possible
B. To arrange induction between 41–42 weeks and discuss membrane sweep
C. To arrange induction with amniotomy at 41 weeks
D. To continue expectant management even after 42 weeks with fetal surveillance until labour commences
E. To observe for 10 days and call again if the mother had not delivered

121 A gravida 2 Para 1, booked for low-risk midwifery care presents at 38 weeks with diminished fetal movements for 48 hours. The fetal heart rate was undetectable and sadly, intrauterine fetal death was confirmed with an ultrasound scan. The mother would prefer to go home and return 24 hours later for induction after arranging childcare for her other child. Her blood group is B RhD negative.

What would you advice?

A. Advice 200 mg of mifepristone and then allow to go home
B. Advice a Kleihauer test and administer anti-RhD gamma globulin and allow to go home
C. Advice Kleihauer test to detect feto-maternal haemorrhage and allow to go home
D. Advice against going home
E. Allow her to go home

122 A British born primigravida with an uncomplicated pregnancy at 22 weeks gestation, needs to travel to sub-Saharan Africa for a family emergency and is expected to spend up to a month in Nigeria.

She wishes to know about the risk of contracting malaria.

What is her risk during a 1-month stay without chemoprophylaxis?

A. 1:5000

B. 1:2500

C. 1:500

D. 1:50

E. 1:20

123 A primigravida is seen in the antenatal clinic. A routine mid trimester anomaly scan at 20 weeks reveals an anterior placenta covering the os.

What is the most appropriate management?

A. Arrange a colour flow doppler scan

B. Arrange an MRI as soon as possible

C. Arrange a transvaginal scan immediately as it will reclassify unto 60% of the cases

D. Reassure the mother and arrange a repeat scan for placental localisation at 36 weeks

E. Reassure the mother that there is no need for any further investigations as the placenta will migrate upward as the pregnancy progresses

124 A gravida 3 Para 2 is diagnosed with an anterior placenta reaching to the os at 20 weeks. She has had 2 previous caesarean sections.

What further investigation would you arrange?

A. Colour flow Doppler scan at 32 weeks

B. MRI scan at 36 weeks

C. No further investigations

D. Transvaginal scan at 32 weeks

E. Ultrasound scan at 36 weeks for placental localisation

125 A 29-year-old primigravida with a low-risk pregnancy attends the obstetric assessment unit with generalzsed pruritus at 34 weeks.

What is the most important investigation to establish a diagnosis of obstetric cholestasis?

A. Bile acids and liver function tests

B. Bile acids and liver function tests with pregnancy-specific reference ranges

C. Coagulation status of the mother

D. Presenting symptoms of the mother

E. Ultrasound estimation of fetal weight

126 A multiparous woman is admitted to a delivery suite at 37 weeks gestation. She has been feeling unwell for the last 48 hours. She gives history of flu-like symptoms with cough, abdominal pain and watery vaginal discharge. Her temperature is 38, pulse 110 per minute, Respiratory rate 24 per minute. You have made a diagnosis of sepsis and antibiotics have been commenced after blood culture. Her serum lactate is 4 mmol/l.

What would be recommended for immediate intravenous fluid resuscitation?

A. Colloid 500 ml
B. Crystalloid 1000 ml
C. Crystalloid 20 ml/kg body weight
D. Crystalloid 40 ml/kg body weight
E. CVP line and fluid as required

127 A primigravida aged 37 is seen at booking. This is a pregnancy following assisted conception. Her BMI is 19 and the ultrasound scan has confirmed a singleton fetus appropriate for the period of gestation.

What is the recommended investigation to identify fetus at risk of SGA age?

A. 2-weekly liquor volume and uterine artery Doppler from 26 weeks
B. 3-weekly serial ultrasound scan for growth and estimated fetal weight from 28 week onwards
C. Detailed anomaly scan to be performed by a fetal medicine specialist at 20 weeks to look for fetal echogenic bowel
D. Growth scans at 28 and 34 weeks
E. Uterine artery Doppler at 20–24 weeks

128 A 40-year-old primigravida is seen in the antenatal clinic with a twin pregnancy conceived through IVF. Gestation is 11 + 6 days and the ultrasound scan has confirmed DCDA twins appropriate for the gestation with normal nuchal thickening.

What is the appropriate monitoring to detect growth discordance?

A. Growth scans at 28 and 34 weeks
B. Serial growth scans every 2 weeks from 20 weeks
C. Serial growth scans with fetal weight estimation every 2 weeks from 16 weeks
D. Serial growth scans with fetal weight estimation every 3–4 weeks from 20 weeks
E. Symphysio-fundal measurement

129 A 38-year-old gravida 3 Para 2 is admitted at 32 week gestation feeling unwell. She has been gradually becoming more anxious through the day with cough and chest pain, which was worse during inspiration. Observations are as follows:

Temperature 37.2 °C, Pulse 110 per minute, BP 98/60, RR 24 per minute and blood gases reveal mild respiratory alkalosis.

What is the most appropriate management plan?

A. Perform an urgent chest X-ray and electrocardiogram and commence the patient on therapeutic unfractionated heparin infusion

B. Perform an urgent chest X-ray and electrocardiogram and commence the patient on therapeutic low molecular weight heparin

C. Request a ventilation-perfusion scan to rule out pulmonary embolism

D. Request an urgent computed tomography pulmonary angiogram to rule out pulmonary embolism

E. Take blood cultures and start the patient on intravenous antibiotics

130 A 37-year-old primigravida weighing 102 kg (BMI 40 kg/m^2) is seen in an antenatal clinic for booking. She conceived via assisted conception following a long period of subfertility. Ultrasound has confirmed a dichorionic diamniotic twin pregnancy of 11 + 5 days gestation.

What is the best practice with regard to reducing maternal risk of venous thromboembolism?

A. Advise compression stockings and mobilisation throughout pregnancy

B. Commence 75 mg of Aspirin per day and advice good hydration and mobilisation

C. Consider and advise low molecular weight heparin – Enoxaparin 40 mg per day throughout pregnancy

D. Consider and advise low molecular weight heparin – Enoxaparin 60 mg per day throughout pregnancy

E. Consider and advise unfractionated heparin daily throughout pregnancy

Module 9

Maternal Medicine

131 A woman with chronic essential hypertension was converted from Lisinopril to methyldopa in a preconception counselling clinic.

The pregnancy was uncomplicated and she delivered spontaneously at term.

At what stage postnatally should the antihypertensive medication be switched back to Lisinopril?

A. 2 days

B. 7 days

C. 14 days

D. 6 weeks

E. 12 weeks

132 A 32-year-old woman primigravida who is 34 weeks pregnant attends the antenatal clinic complaining of severe itching.

Serum bile acids are found to be elevated and she is diagnosed with obstetric cholestasis.

What is the most effective medication to improve her itching?

A. Activated charcoal

B. Chlorphenamine

C. Colestyramine

D. S-adenosyl methionine

E. Ursodeoxycholic acid

133 What is the main contraindication to the use of antenatal corticosteroids?

A. Chorioamnionitis

B. Cushing's syndrome

C. Diabetes mellitus

D. Multiple pregnancy

E. Systemic infection

134 In the recent MBRRACE-UK report (2014), what was the leading overall single cause of maternal death?

A. Cardiac disease

B. Haemorrhage

C. Sepsis

D. Suicide

E. Thromboembolism

135 An anaesthetist is asked to assist with the insertion of an intravenous cannula prior to the commencement of a Syntocinon infusion in labour.

The cannula is inserted successfully, but shortly after it was flushed through as the woman starts to have convulsions and becomes hypotensive and bradycardic.

The syringes on the trolley are unlabeled and the anaesthetist suspects he may have flushed the cannula with a local anaesthetic solution.

What is the appropriate management of her collapse?

A. Activated charcoal orally

B. Calcium gluconate 10% IV

C. Intralipid 20% infusion

D. Magnesium sulphate 20% IV

E. Potassium chloride 10% IV

136 A 32-year-old woman with known HIV-1 infection is being seen in antenatal clinic in her first pregnancy. Her viral load is <50 copies/ml at 36 weeks gestation and she wishes to have further pregnancies in the future.

What is the most significant intervention to reduce mother to child transmission?

A. Avoiding invasive procedures during delivery

B. Elective caesarean section at term

C. Exclusive replacement feeding of the baby

D. Initiation of antiretroviral therapy during pregnancy

E. Mixed feeding of the baby

137 Prior to the development of highly active antiretroviral therapy (HAART), elective caesarean section was the standard mode of delivery to reduce intrapartum mother to child transmission of HIV.

At what viral load should caesarean section be considered with present HAART management?

A. 0–50 copies/ml

B. 50–400 copies/ml

C. 400–500 copies/ml

D. 500–600 copies/ml

E. 600–700 copies/ml

138 With the present multidisciplinary management of HIV in pregnancy using HAART, what is the rate of mother to child transmission of HIV in the United Kingdom?

A. 0.3%

B. 0.7%

C. 1.5%

D. 3%

E. 6%

139 A woman who is HIV positive attends antenatal clinic at 36 weeks gestation. She has an uncomplicated pregnancy.

At what plasma viral load could vaginal delivery be recommended?

A. Less than 50 HIV RNA copies/ml

B. Less than 100 HIV RNA copies/ml

C. Less than 150 HIV RNA copies/ml

D. Less than 200 HIV RNA copies/ml

E. Less than 250 HIV RNA copies/ml

140 A 29-year-old primigravida attends her booking visit at 12 + 2 days. An ultrasound scan has confirmed a live fetus appropriate for the period of gestation. She is known to be HIV positive and is not in need of treatment for her own health, with a viral load of >35,000 copies/ml and is very keen for a vaginal delivery.

What is the most appropriate intervention with regards to reducing the risk of neonatal transmission of HIV?

A. Advise against vaginal delivery and recommend elective LSCS at 38 weeks

B. Initiate cART at the beginning of second trimester weeks and to be discontinued at delivery

C. Initiate cART immediately and continued for 6 weeks postpartum

D. Initiate zidovudine monotherapy immediately and continue for 6 weeks postpartum

E. Initiate zidovudine monotherapy immediately and discontinue at delivery

141 A 29-year-old gravida 2 para 1 is admitted with history of preterm prelabour rupture of membranes at 31 + 5 weeks gestation of 4 hours duration. She is a known HIV patient with a low viral load and had been commenced on HAART at 22 weeks. Her viral load at 28 weeks was <50 copies/ml. On admission, she is apyrexial, vital signs are within normal limits and the CTG is reassuring.

What is the most appropriate immediate management with regard to delivery?

A. Undertake genital infection screen, rapid testing for current viral load, administer steroids and oral erythromycin and arrange MDT consultation

B. Undertake genital infection screen, rapid testing of current viral load, commence broad-spectrum antibiotics and arrange for category 1 LSCS

C. Undertake genital infection screen, rapid testing of current viral load, commence broad-spectrum antibiotic and arrange for category 2 LSCS

D. Undertake genital infection screen, rapid testing of current viral load, commence broad-spectrum antibiotics and arrange for category 3 LSCS

E. Undertake genital infection screen and rapid testing for current viral load, administer steroids and induce labour after 48 hours

142 A 29-year-old gravida 2 para 1 is seen in an antenatal clinic at 37 weeks for the first time. She has transferred her booking from another region, where she had been diagnosed as HIV positive. Her viral load is 1000 copies/ml. She does not need treatment for her own health and was started on zidovudine monotherapy at the previous hospital. Her previous delivery was spontaneous vaginal delivery with no complications.

What is the most appropriate management plan for delivery?

A. Advise to continue zidovudine therapy and arrange elective caesarean at 38 weeks with intravenous zidovudine cover for delivery to be discontinued at delivery

B. Advise to continue zidovudine therapy and arrange elective caesarean at 38 weeks with intravenous cover for delivery and change over to cART after delivery

C. Advise to continue zidovudine therapy and await spontaneous labour with intravenous zidovudine cover during labour and discontinue at delivery

D. Stop zidovudine and initiate cART and arrange for elective caesarean section at 38 weeks and discontinue treatment at delivery

E. Stop zidovudine and initiate cART and await spontaneous labour and discontinue treatment at delivery

143 A young primigravida attends assessment unit at 32 weeks gestation following an assessment of raised blood pressure by the community midwife. Urine protein: creatinine ratio is 32 mg/mmol and her blood pressure is 152/102 mmHg.

What is the most appropriate management plan?

A. Admit and commence antihypertensive treatment

B. Admit for observation with 6-hourly blood pressure monitoring and daily protein: creatinine ratio

C. Admit for observation

D. Discharge back to community midwife with advice for blood pressure and automated reagent-strip test for proteinuria twice weekly

E. Discharge back to community midwife with advice for blood pressure and urine protein: creatinine ratio on a daily basis

144 A primigravida with a BMI of 34 kg/m^2 presents at 21 weeks gestation with severe throbbing headache and vomiting. She gives a history of similar headaches in the past. On examination, her blood pressure is found to be normal with no proteinuria and the deep tendon reflexes are normal. A neurological review is arranged as there are no localising neurological signs except mild bilateral sixth nerve paresis.

What is the most likely diagnosis?

A. Benign idiopathic intracranial hypertension

B. Depression

C. Migraine

D. Pre-eclampsia

E. Space occupying lesion

145 A primigravida has been brought to the Accident and Emergency department following a road traffic accident at 32 weeks gestation. The obstetric registrar is summoned urgently. On arrival she learns that CPR had been commenced 3 minutes earlier following a diagnosis of cardiac arrest and pulseless electrical activity.

What is the most appropriate initial action for an ST5 trainee?

A. Advise ALS algorithm

B. Advise Dexamethasone for fetal lung maturity

C. Arrange transfer to delivery suite for category 1 caesarean section

D. Call the consultant

E. Prepare and commence caesarean section with the aim to achieve delivery within 5 minutes of maternal collapse

146 A primigravida aged 30 attends antenatal clinic at 34 weeks gestation. She is known to have mild bipolar disorder but has not required any medication prior to pregnancy. Her mother suffers from bipolar disorder and takes lithium. During the visit she reports increasing anxiety, depression and self-neglect.

To which health professional should this patient be referred?

A. Community midwife

B. Consultant Obstetrician

C. General Practitioner for appropriate medications

D. General Practitioner with advice for CPN Support

E. Specialised perinatal mental health services or general psychiatry services as available

147 A 39-year-old Type 2 diabetic of Asian origin presents with an acute onset of epigastric pain, chest pain and breathlessness at 30 weeks gestation. She is gravida 5 Para 4 (four normal vaginal deliveries), and has a BMI of 41 kg/m². This was an unplanned pregnancy. Her diabetes is poorly controlled and her haemoglobin was 85 g/1 at 28 weeks. She is on oral iron and there is history of familial hyperlipidemia.

What is the most likely working diagnosis for this mother?
   A. Acute myocardial infarction (AMI)
   B. Chest infection
   C. Pulmonary embolism
   D. Pulmonary edema
   E. Rib flaring/musculoskeletal pain

148 A 32-year-old primigravida is admitted in spontaneous early labour at 39 + 2 weeks. She is a known asthmatic and has had repeated admissions in this pregnancy with acute exacerbations of asthma. The previous admission had been at 36 weeks gestation when she was commenced on oral prednisolone 7.5 mg/day in view of persistent poor asthmatic control.

What is the most appropriate intervention to maintain asthma control in labour?
   A. 100 mg of parenteral hydrocortisone 6–8 hourly during labour
   B. Continuous oxygen by face mask
   C. Deliver by caesarean section
   D. Refer to a respiratory physician
   E. Regular inhaled long-acting Beta 2 agonist along with her current medications

149 A 29-year-old primigravida with a low-risk pregnancy attends the obstetric assessment unit with generalised pruritus at 34 weeks gestation. Laboratory results reveal bile acids of 16 mmol/l with normal Liver Function Tests (LFT) and you have established a diagnosis of Obstetric Cholestasis.

What is considered to be the best practice with regard to further antenatal care?
   A. Reassure and continue with midwifery care along with weekly Bile acid and LFT estimation
   B. Reassure and continue with midwifery care and arrange induction of labour at 37–38 weeks
   C. Reassure and transfer booking to consultant-led care
   D. Review mother in the assessment unit, discuss increased risk of stillbirth and arrange induction of labour at 37–38 weeks
   E. Transfer booking to consultant-led care and arrange a clinic review with repeat bile acid and LFT estimation

150 An 18-year-old primigravida is seen in the antenatal clinic for booking at 8 weeks gestation. She is known to have sickle cell disease and her partner is known to have normal haemoglobin. She has recently arrived from Nigeria and has not taken any vitamin supplements so far.

What is the most important vitamin supplement during pregnancy?

A. Folic acid 1 mg immediately for throughout pregnancy
B. Folic acid 400 µg immediately for throughout pregnancy
C. Folic acid 400 µg immediately until 12 weeks gestation
D. Folic acid 5 mg immediately for throughout pregnancy
E. Folic acid 5 mg immediately until 12 weeks gestation

151 An 18-year-old primigravida, a recent immigrant from West Africa is admitted at 30 weeks gestation with severe pain in her hips. A diagnosis of acute painful sickle cell crisis has been made.

What is the most important immediate management?

A. Admission and rapid assessment followed by morphine for pain relief
B. Admission and rapid assessment followed by non-steroidal anti-inflammatory drugs
C. Admission and rapid assessment followed by oxygen and hydration without any analgesics
D. Admission and rapid assessment followed by Pethidine for pain relief
E. Observation and discharge home with Codeine and paracetamol

152 A 31-year-old primigravida presents for booking at 10 weeks. She is known to be hypothyroid and is on Levothyroxine 75 µg. She is complaining of feeling tired and lethargic and her TSH is 6.5 mU/ml.

What would be the target TSH level at this gestation to indicate optimal control?

A. 0.1–2.5 mU/ml
B. 0.5–3.5 mU/m
C. 4.5 mU/ml is satisfactory
D. Just below 4.5 mU/ml
E. Obtain advice from an Endocrine Specialist

153 A 38-year-old pregnant woman with obesity and Type 2 diabetes presents with chest pain at 28 weeks gestation. Which is the blood marker of choice for diagnosis of AMI in pregnancy?
A. Creatine kinase isoenzyme MB
B. C-reactive protein
C. Lactate dehydrogenase
D. Myoglobin
E. Troponin

154 Following diagnosis of AMI in pregnancy, which medication should not be used in the acute phase?
A. Aspirin
B. Labetalol
C. Low molecular weight heparin
D. Nifedipine
E. Unfractionated heparin

155 What is the approximate incidence of overt hypothyroidism in pregnancy?
A. 0.1%
B. 0.5%
C. 1.0%
D. 2.0%
E. 2.5%

156 A 41-year-old woman has an oral glucose tolerance test (OGTT) at 28 weeks gestation in her fourth pregnancy. The results are as follows:

Fasting plasma glucose: 5.8 mmol/l
2 hour plasma glucose: 7.4 mmol/l

What is the correct diagnosis?
A. Impaired glucose tolerance
B. Gestational diabetes
C. Maturity onset diabetes of the young (MODY)
D. Normal glycemic control
E. Type 2 diabetes

157 A 30-year-old woman is diagnosed with gestational diabetes following an oral glucose tolerance test (OGGT) at 26 weeks gestation in her first pregnancy. Her fasting blood glucose is 7.2 mmol/l. What is the appropriate management?
A. Dietary modification alone
B. Dietary modification and exercise
C. Glibenclamide
D. Insulin
E. Metformin

158 A 20-year-old woman with Type 1 diabetes presents at 32 weeks gestation in her first pregnancy with regular painful contractions, a closed cervix and a positive fetal fibronectin test. What is the most appropriate management plan?
   A. Antenatal steroids
   B. Antenatal steroids and additional insulin
   C. Antenatal steroids and tocolysis with atosiban
   D. Antenatal steroids, additional insulin and tocolysis with atosiban
   E. Tocolysis with atosiban

159 What is the prevalence of asthma in pregnant women?
   A. 0.1–0.4%
   B. 0.5–1%
   C. 2–3%
   D. 4–12%
   E. 14–20%

160 For women with severe asthma, in what proportion does disease further deteriorate during pregnancy?
   A. 10%
   B. 30%
   C. 40%
   D. 50%
   E. 60%

161 For which group of women is vitamin K supplementation advised in the last month of pregnancy?
   A. Women taking anti-epileptic drugs
   B. Women with two or more risk factors for pre-eclampsia
   C. Women with a body mass index (BMI) >35
   D. Women with liver disease
   E. Women with pre-existing diabetes

162 A woman with a BMI of 40 whose epilepsy is well controlled on anti-epileptic drugs (AEDs) attends for a booking appointment with the community midwife at 10 weeks gestation. Which combination of vitamin supplements should she be advised to take?
   A. Folic acid 400 mcg and vitamin D 10 mcg
   B. Folic acid 400 mcg and vitamin K 10 mg
   C. Folic acid 5 mg and vitamin C 70 mg
   D. Folic acid 5 mg and vitamin D 10 mcg
   E. Vitamin D 10 mcg and vitamin C 70 mg

163 A woman who is taking antipsychotic medication is contemplating pregnancy.

Why is Lithium not the drug of choice ?

A. Risk of cardiac defects in the fetus

B. Risk of constipation in the fetus

C. Risk of gestational diabetes

D. Risk of maternal hypertension

E. Possible risk of neonatal persistent pulmonary hypertension

164 A woman is recently diagnosed with gestational diabetes. A programme of exercise and dietary change is initiated. What is the likelihood of her needing further treatment with an oral hypoglycemic agent or insulin therapy in this pregnancy?

A. 1–2%

B. 10–20%

C. 30–40%

D. 80%+

E. 90%+

165 A woman attends the perimental health antenatal clinic at 8 weeks of gestation. She wishes to stop her lithium therapy with the support of her psychiatrist and seeks advice.

What should be the recommended action after fully counselling the patient?

A. Immediately stop lithium therapy due to its high teratogenic risks

B. Mandatory to continue in pregnancy due to the high risk of mania

C. Stop gradually over the next 4 weeks to reduce the risk of mania

D. Stop immediately but convert to Carbamazepine

E. Stop only if patient agrees to accept an additional antipsychotic treatment

166 A woman attends clinic for preconceptual counselling after previously being treated for breast carcinoma. She is planning a pregnancy. How long after completion of the treatment is it recommended to wait before conceiving?

A. 1 month

B. 6 months

C. 1 year

D. 2 years

E. 3 years

167 A primagravida who is otherwise fit and well, sadly, has a stillbirth at 38 weeks of gestation.

In what proportion of cases is there no identifiable cause?

A. Almost 10% of cases

B. Almost 30% of cases

C. Almost 50% of cases

D. Almost 70% of cases

E. Almost 90% of cases

168 A woman with known sickle cell trait attends an antenatal booking clinic.

What antenatal complication is significantly more common compared to uncomplicated pregnancies?

A. Chest infection

B. Intrauterine growth restriction

C. Major postpartum haemorrhage

D. Placental abruption

E. Urinary tract infection

169 A woman attends the antenatal clinic in a wheel chair with a known long-term traumatic spinal cord injury.

At what level of spinal injury and above would you be concerned about the occurrence of autonomic dysreflexia?

A. T6

B. T10

C. T12

D. L3

E. L5

170 A 25-year-old woman presents at 12 weeks gestation. Four years earlier she presented with a deep vein thrombosis after fracturing her femur and undergoing a major orthopaedic operation. Her thrombophilia screen result is negative, she has no family history of thrombosis and she has a body mass index of 23 kg/m^2.

What thromboprophylaxis should be offered to this woman?

A. 6 weeks of low molecular weight heparin postnatal

B. Aspirin antenatally and 6 week of low molecular weight heparin postnatal

C. Immediate treatment of low molecular weight heparin until 37 weeks of gestation

D. Immediate treatment of low molecular weight heparin until 6 weeks postpartum

E. Start low molecular weight heparin at 28 weeks until 6 weeks postpartum

Module 10

Management of Labour

171 A 32-year-old gravida 2 Para 1 has been transferred from a midwifery-led unit for lack of progress in labour at 4 cm. Her previous baby weighed 3100 g and was a normal delivery at 38 weeks gestation. On admission, her observations are normal and the cardiotocography (CTG) was reassuring. The midwife who examined her has diagnosed a complete breech presentation and this is confirmed on scan. The woman is very keen to have a vaginal delivery and decision has been taken to allow labour to continue. After 2 hours, there is no progress in labour and the CTG has become suspicious.

What is the most appropriate action?
A. Advice emergency caesarean section
B. Augment labour with syntocinon
C. Continue observation for one hour
D. Discuss ECV with the mother
E. Perform fetal blood sampling

172 A Gravida 4 Para 3 (three normal deliveries at term) is admitted in preterm labour at 36 + 5 days. She is known to have polyhydramnios but relevant antenatal investigations have been normal. An ultrasound scan at 36 weeks gestation had revealed the estimated fetal weight to be just below the 10th centile on a customized growth chart.

On examination, the cervix was 4 cm dilated with intact membranes and a high presenting part. Five minutes after admission there is spontaneous rupture of membranes and the CTG shows fetal bradycardia.

Part 2 MRCOG: Single Best Answer Questions, First Edition.
Andrew Sizer, Chandrika Balachandar, Nibedan Biswas, Richard Foon,
Anthony Griffiths, Sheena Hodgett, Banchhita Sahu and Martyn Underwood.
© 2016 John Wiley & Sons, Ltd. Published 2016 by John Wiley & Sons, Ltd.

What needs to be excluded by a prompt vaginal examination?

A. Amniotic fluid embolism

B. Breech presentation

C. Cord prolapse

D. Placental abruption

E. Shoulder/arm prolapse

173 A primigravida who is a Type 1 diabetic is admitted in labour at 37 + 2 weeks gestation. The midwife has commenced sliding scale insulin infusion.

Between which values should the capillary blood glucose be maintained during labour?

A. 3 and 8 mmol/l

B. 3.5 and 5.9 mmol/l

C. 4 and 7 mmol/l

D. 5 and 9 mmol/l

E. 6 and 8 mmol/l

174 A gravida 3 Para 2 (both full term normal deliveries) is admitted at term with confirmed rupture of membranes and labour has been augmented with syntocinon. The woman has suffered from recurrent herpes during pregnancy and is noted to have recurrent genital lesions on admission. At 4–5 cm dilatation, the liquor is noted to have grade II meconium and the CTG has been suspicious for the last 40 minutes.

What is the most appropriate action at this stage?

A. To advise emergency caesarean section to expedite delivery

B. To commence intravenous acyclovir

C. To perform fetal blood sample to assess the acid base status of the baby

D. To review the syntocinon and increase the dose to expedite delivery

E. To stop the syntocinon and advice to continue observation

175 You are working in an Obstetric unit with level 2 Neonatal care facilities. A primigravida is admitted to the delivery suite at 32 weeks gestation with painful contractions and confirmed preterm prelabour rupture of membranes (PROM). She is pyrexial with a temperature of 38°C and a pulse of 108/minute. CTG confirms regular contractions and there is fetal tachycardia of 170 bpm with good variability. A speculum examination had shown the cervix to be 2–3 cm dilated. Two weeks prior to this admission the woman had been seen in the day assessment unit with threatened preterm labour and had received two doses of dexamethasone.
What is the most appropriate management?
- **A.** Commence antibiotics after septic screen and allow labour to continue with continuous electronic fetal monitoring and inform neonatal unit
- **B.** Commence antibiotics and arrange in utero transfer to a level 3 neonatal unit
- **C.** Commence tocolysis and arrange in utero transfer to a level 3 neonatal unit
- **D.** Repeat dexamethasone, along with tocolysis and inform neonatal unit
- **E.** Repeat dexamethasone, commence antibiotics and prepare for emergency caesarean section

176 What type of headache is associated with a dural puncture?
- **A.** Fronto–occipital location
- **B.** Occipital location
- **C.** Temporal location
- **D.** Temporal with non-focal neurology
- **E.** Thunderclap

177 A 24-year-old with a known hypersensitivity reaction to penicillin presents at 36 weeks of gestation in established labour. A high vaginal swab in this pregnancy has noted a growth of group B streptococcus. What intrapartum antibiotic prophylaxis would you offer?
- **A.** Benzyl penicillin
- **B.** Ceftriaxone
- **C.** Clindamycin
- **D.** Co-amoxiclav
- **E.** Erythromycin

178 A 25-year-old woman with no known drug allergies presents in early labour with ruptured membranes at 39 weeks gestation. She received intrapartum antibiotic prophylaxis (IAP) in her first labour following the identification of group B streptococcus (GBS) bacteriuria during pregnancy. She had a healthy baby with no neonatal problems. What is the most appropriate management?

A. IAP with intravenous ampicillin

B. IAP with intravenous benzylpenicillin

C. IAP with intravenous clindamycin

D. IAP with intravenous erythromycin

E. No intrapartum antibiotic prophylaxis

179 When considering local regimens for intrapartum antibiotic pro-phylaxis (IAP), what proportion of neonatal infection developing within 48 hours of birth in the United Kingdom is caused by group B streptococcus (GBS)?

A. 30%

B. 40%

C. 50%

D. 60%

E. 70%

180 A 34-year-old woman presents in spontaneous labour at 38 weeks gestation in her second pregnancy, having had a previous prelabour caesarean section for breech presentation. In the first stage of labour, she develops continuous lower abdominal pain and a tachycardia. The fetal heart rate becomes bradycardic. She is delivered by urgent (category1) caesarean section and uterine rupture is confirmed. What is the risk of perinatal mortality?

A. 0.2%

B. 0.5%

C. 1%

D. 2%

E. 5%

181 A 42-year-old woman is 39 weeks gestation in her second pregnancy having had a prior emergency caesarean section for fetal distress three years earlier. She is keen to give birth vaginally but is requesting induction of labour because of concerns regarding the increased risk of perinatal mortality associated with her age.

What is the most appropriate method of induction to minimise the risk of uterine rupture in labour?

    A. Amniotomy and oxytocin
    B. Dinoprostone
    C. Misoprostol
    D. Oxytocin alone
    E. Transcervical Foley catheter

182 What is the incidence of cord prolapse with breech presentation?

    A. 0.1%
    B. 0.2%
    C. 0.6%
    D. 1%
    E. 2%

183 When umbilical cord prolapse occurs in the community setting, what is the increase in risk of perinatal mortality?

    A. 2 times
    B. 4 times
    C. 6 times
    D. 8 times
    E. 10 times

184 In otherwise uncomplicated preterm labour, evidence suggests that the use of tocolysis delays delivery. By how long does it delay delivery?

    A. 24 hours
    B. 48 hours
    C. 72 hours
    D. 7 days
    E. 14 days

185 Which tocolytic drug is comparably effective and has a similar incidence of maternal side effects to Atosiban when used to suppress preterm labour?

    A. Glyceryl trinitrate
    B. Indomethacin
    C. Magnesium sulphate
    D. Nifedipine
    E. Terbutaline

186 A 25-year-old woman with no known drug allergies presents in early labour at 37 weeks gestation in her first pregnancy. Her membranes ruptured an hour prior to admission. Her temperature is 38.1° C, she is clinically well and the fetal heart rate is normal. What is the most appropriate management?

A. Category 1 caesarean section
B. Category 2 caesarean section
C. Treatment with intravenous antibiotics including benzylpenicillin
D. Treatment with intravenous antibiotics including erythromycin
E. Treatment with intravenous paracetamol and rechecking temperature in 2 hours

187 A 20-year-old woman presents at 40 weeks gestation in her first pregnancy with irregular contractions, offensive vaginal discharge and reduced fetal movements. She has a temperature of 39.2 °C and a tachycardia. On examination, the cervix is effaced and 4 cm dilated and membranes are absent. The fetal heart rate is 170 bpm. Broad spectrum antibiotics are administered after taking blood cultures. What is the most appropriate subsequent management?

A. Augmentation of labour with oxytocin
B. Category 2 caesarean section with general anaesthesia (GA)
C. Category 2 caesarean section with spinal anaesthesia
D. Epidural analgesia and fetal blood sampling (FBS)
E. Reassess progress in 4 hours

188 A 24-year-old woman with sickle cell disease is admitted for induction of labour at 38 weeks gestation in her first pregnancy that is otherwise uncomplicated. Three hours after commencement of intravenous oxytocin, her oxygen saturation drops to 93%. What is the most appropriate immediate management?

A. Administer oxygen therapy and check arterial blood gases
B. Administer oxygen therapy and intravenous antibiotics
C. Category 1 caesarean section with general anaesthesia (GA)
D. Category 2 caesarean section with regional analgesia
E. Stop the oxytocin infusion

189 A 19-year-old woman is admitted at 34 weeks and 4 days gestation in her second pregnancy with spontaneous rupture of membranes and painful uterine contractions. Her first pregnancy resulted in a spontaneous preterm birth at 32 weeks gestation. On examination, the cervix is fully effaced and 6 cm dilated. What is the most appropriate treatment?
A. Atosiban 6.75 mg intravenously
B. Benzylpenicillin 1.2 g intravenously
C. Betamethasone 12 mg intramuscularly
D. Nifedipine 20 mg orally
E. Pethidine 100 mg intramuscularly

190 A 31-year-old woman with well-controlled Type 1 diabetes is admitted for induction of labour at 38 weeks gestation in her second pregnancy having had a previous spontaneous normal birth at 36 weeks gestation. After vaginal examination confirms that she is 6 cm dilated, her blood sugar drops to 3.5 mmol/l and she has no symptoms of hypoglycemia.
What is the most appropriate management?
A. Allow light diet and recheck blood sugar after one hour
B. Commence intravenous dextrose and insulin infusion
C. Give intramuscular glucagon and recheck blood sugar after one hour
D. Give oral glucose gel and recheck blood sugar after one hour
E. Recheck blood sugar after 30 minutes

191 What percentage of women with PROM at term will go into labour within the next 24 hours?
A. 40%
B. 50%
C. 60%
D. 70%
E. 75%

192 A low-risk 25-year-old woman at 40 weeks gestation is labouring in the birthing pool in her local midwifery-led unit. She is 8 cm dilated when her midwife checks the temperature of the water, which is 37.7 °C. What is the most appropriate immediate management?
A. Add cold water to the birthing pool
B. Ask her to get out of the pool temporarily
C. Encourage her to drink more water
D. Give oral paracetamol 1 g
E. Recheck the water temperature in 30 minutes

193 A low-risk 34-year-old woman in her second pregnancy is admitted in spontaneous labour at 39 weeks gestation. Her cervix is effaced and 5 cm dilated with membranes intact on admission. She is examined again four hours later and is 6 cm dilated; she consents to artificial rupture of membranes (ARM), liquor is clear.
What is the most appropriate method of fetal monitoring?
A. CTG for 20 minutes followed by intermittent auscultation
B. Continuous CTG with abdominal transducer
C. Continuous CTG with fetal scalp electrode
D. CTG for 40 minutes followed by intermittent auscultation
E. Intermittent auscultation

194 What proportion of intrapartum CTG with reduced fetal heart rate baseline variability and late decelerations results in moderate to severe cerebral palsy in children?
A. 0.1%
B. 0.2%
C. 0.5%
D. 1%
E. 1.5%

195 When evaluated as an adjunct to CTG for intrapartum fetal monitoring, of which outcome has STAN (ST analysis) been shown to reduce incidence?
A. Caesarean section
B. Low Apgar scores
C. Neonatal encephalopathy
D. Operative vaginal delivery
E. Severe fetal metabolic acidosis

Module 11

Management of Delivery

196 What is the risk of neonatal herpes infection in a woman with recurrent genital HSV infection if lesions are present at the time of vaginal delivery?
A. 0–3%
B. 10–13%
C. 20–23%
D. 30–33%
E. 40–43%

197 A primigravida is in spontaneous preterm labour at 35 + 1 weeks of gestation. She has progressed satisfactorily in labour and has been pushing for ten minutes. Fifteen minutes prior to pushing, a fetal blood sampling had been performed due to a suspicious CTG and the result was normal. You have been asked to attend as the CTG shows prolonged bradycardia. You are not able to feel the fetal head abdominally and the vertex is at +2 station and is less than 45 degrees from the occipito-anterior position.
What is the most appropriate course of action?
A. Expedite delivery by performing a caesarean section
B. Expedite delivery with low mid-cavity forceps
C. Expedite delivery with rotational forceps
D. Expedite delivery with Ventouse
E. Repeat fetal blood sampling

198 A gravida 3 Para 2 is diagnosed with anterior placenta reaching to the os at 20 weeks gestation. She has had 2 previous caesarean sections. Further imaging with colour flow doppler at 32 weeks has confirmed major placenta praevia and placenta accreta.
What would be the recommendation for delivery?
A. Category 3 caesarean section as soon as possible
B. Elective caesarean section at 36–37 weeks
C. Elective caesarean section at 38 weeks
D. Elective caesarean section at 39 weeks
E. Elective caesarean section at term

199 Sequential use of instruments increases neonatal trauma.
By what factor is the incidence of subdural and intracranial haemorrhage increased in this situation?
A. 1.5 times
B. 2–3 times
C. 3–4 times
D. Up to 5 times
E. 10 times

200 An emergency buzzer has been activated for shoulder dystocia. You are instructing two junior midwives to assist you in delivery with McRoberts' maneuvre.
What would you ask them to do?
A. Hyperflex and adduct maternal thighs onto her abdomen
B. Hyperflex and adduct maternal thighs on her abdomen
C. Perform an episiotomy
D. Place the mother in a lithotomy position
E. Provide fundal pressure

201 The hospital blood transfusion committee requires guidance with regard to the use of cell salvage in Obstetrics.
On which occasions of caesarean section is cell salvage recommended?
A. Only for women who reject the use of blood products
B. When the intra-operative blood loss is anticipated to be greater than 1000 ml
C. When the intra-operative blood loss is anticipated to be greater than 1500 ml
D. When there is a high risk of platelet dysfunction
E. When there is an established coagulopathy

202 In the case of a massive obstetric haemorrhage, above what level should fibrinogen be maintained?

A. 0.5 g/l

B. 1 g/l

C. 2 g/l

D. 5 g/l

E. 10 g/l

203 You are asked to assess a woman's perineum after a vaginal delivery. There is an extensive tear disrupting the superficial muscle and 70 % of the external anal sphincter. There is no disruption of the internal anal sphincter. How would you classify this perineal trauma?

A. Second degree tear

B. 3a tear

C. 3b tear

D. 3c tear

E. Fourth degree tear

204 A 40-year-old woman is diagnosed with acute myocardial infarction (AMI) at 36 weeks gestation in her second pregnancy, she is clinically stable. She had a previous normal vaginal delivery at term in her local hospital.

What is the most appropriate plan for timing and mode of delivery?

A. Antenatal steroids and delivery by elective caesarean section in her local hospital

B. Await spontaneous labour and delivery in her local hospital

C. Immediate transfer to a high risk obstetric unit and urgent delivery by caesarean section

D. Induction of labour at 38–39 weeks gestation in a high risk obstetric unit with intensive care expertise

E. Induction of labour in her local hospital at 37 weeks gestation

205 A 28-year-old woman presents in spontaneous labour at 41 weeks gestation with a cephalic presentation in her third pregnancy having had two previous normal births. At the onset of the second stage, she ruptures her membranes and the fetal heart rate decelerates. Vaginal examination confirms umbilical cord prolapse with the fetal head in direct occipito-anterior position below the level of the ischial spines.

What is the optimal management?

A. Anticipation of normal delivery and encouragement to push

B. Bladder filling to displace the fetal head and replacement of the prolapsed umbilical cord

C. Category 1 caesarean section under general anaesthesia

D. Digital elevation of the fetal head and category 2 caesarean section with regional anaesthesia

E. Immediate operative vaginal delivery with ventouse extraction

206 A 40-year-old woman with Type 2 diabetes is admitted for induction of labour at 38 weeks gestation in her third pregnancy having had two previous spontaneous normal births. She has epidural analgesia for pain relief and her labour is uncomplicated until shoulder dystocia is diagnosed after delivery of the fetal head. Additional help is summoned but the shoulders cannot be delivered with axial traction and suprapubic pressure in McRoberts' position.

What is the most appropriate subsequent management?

A. Adopt 'all fours' position

B. Attempt delivery of the posterior arm

C. Attempt Zavanelli maneuvre

D. Downward traction

E. Fundal pressure

207 A low-risk 27-year-old woman is induced at 41+ 5 weeks gestation in her second pregnancy, having had a previous ventouse delivery for fetal distress. She has epidural analgesia for pain relief in labour. Following confirmation of full cervical dilatation and an hour of passive second stage, she pushes with contractions for 90 minutes without signs of imminent birth. She feels well, her contractions are strong, 4 in 10 minutes and the fetal heart rate is normal.

What is the most appropriate management?

A. Commence intravenous oxytocin

B. Consider operative vaginal delivery after a further 30 minutes, if no change

C. Consider operative vaginal delivery after a further 60 minutes, if no change

D. Discuss operative vaginal delivery immediately

E. Encourage directed pushing in lithotomy position

208 Following a prolonged second stage of labour, a primigravida at term is examined in order to make a decision about operative vaginal delivery.

Abdominal examination indicates that the fetal head is not palpable.

Vaginal examination shows the presenting part to be in a direct occipito-anterior position with a station of +3, and a decision is made to perform a ventouse (vacuum extraction) delivery.

How would you classify this operative vaginal delivery?

A. High

B. Low – rotation of 45° or less

C. Low – rotation of more than 45°

D. Mid

E. Outlet

209 What is the lower limit of gestational age for the use of the vacuum extractor (ventouse)?

A. 32/40

B. 34/40

C. 36/40

D. 38/40

E. 40/40

210 What type of morbidity is <u>less</u> likely to be associated with vacuum extraction than with forceps delivery?

A. Cephalohematoma

B. Low Apgar score at 5 minutes

C. Neonatal jaundice

D. Retinal haemorrhage

E. Vaginal and perineal trauma

Module 12

Postnatal Care

211 A 38-year-old Asian mother has delivered her fourth baby normally. She is a known Type 2 diabetic and was taking Metformin prior to pregnancy for glycemic control. From 32 weeks gestation, Isophane insulin was added twice daily in addition to Metformin to achieve glycemic control. The woman is planning to breast feed. What advice should be given with regard to a hypoglycemic agent in the postnatal period?

   A. Continue all the medications for the first 24 hours after delivery and then resume Metformin as per prepregnancy with monitoring of blood sugar
   B. Stop all medications and follow diet control with monitoring of blood sugar
   C. Stop Insulin and advise Metformin as per prepregnancy with monitoring of blood sugar
   D. Stop Metformin and continue Isophane insulin twice daily until breast feeding has stopped
   E. Stop Metformin and continue Isophane insulin at half the dose used during pregnancy until breastfeeding is stopped

212 A 17-year-old Para 1 is attending for postnatal follow-up 6 weeks after an emergency caesarean section for severe pre-eclampsia and HELLP at 27+ 2 days gestation. The baby was severely growth-restricted and is still in the neonatal unit.
   What is her risk of pre-eclampsia in a future pregnancy?

   A. 13%
   B. 16%
   C. 25%
   D. 45%
   E. 55%

Part 2 MRCOG: Single Best Answer Questions, First Edition.
Andrew Sizer, Chandrika Balachandar, Nibedan Biswas, Richard Foon,
Anthony Griffiths, Sheena Hodgett, Banchhita Sahu and Martyn Underwood.
© 2016 John Wiley & Sons, Ltd. Published 2016 by John Wiley & Sons, Ltd.

213 A woman who is a recent immigrant to the United Kingdom is admitted in labour and delivers rapidly. At delivery, the midwife had noted that the liquor was offensive and appropriate swabs were taken. The mother is also noted to have a low-grade pyrexia and mild tachycardia. Within minutes of antibiotic administration, the mother collapses and anaphylactic shock is diagnosed. An A, B, C, D, E approach has been initiated.

What is the definitive treatment for anaphylaxis?

A. 50 micrograms (0.5 ml) of intra-cardiac 1:10,000 adrenaline

B. 500 micrograms (0.5 ml) of 1:1000 adrenaline intramuscularly

C. 500 micrograms (0.5 ml) of 1:1000 adrenaline intravenously

D. Chlorpheneramine 10 mg intramuscularly

E. Hydrocortisone 200 mg – Intravenously

214 A primigravida aged 30 attends the antenatal clinic for booking. She is known to have Bipolar Disorder and was taking lithium, which was stopped preconceptually due to concerns over fetal toxicity. Her mother is known to have bipolar disorder.

What is her risk of developing postpartum psychosis?

A. 25%

B. 35%

C. 40%

D. 50%

E. 70%

215 A 35-year-old grandmultipara has had a major postpartum haemorrhage (PPH) following a normal delivery. Mechanical and pharmacological measures have failed to control the bleeding. Examination has confirmed that there are no retained placental tissue in the uterine cavity and absence of trauma to genital tract.

What is the most appropriate first-line surgical management?

A. B-Lynch or modified compression sutures

B. Balloon tamponade

C. Ligation of internal iliac artery

D. Postpartum hysterectomy

E. Selective arterial embolisation

216 Active management of the third stage of labour reduces the risk of PPH.

By what proportion is the risk of PPH reduced by prophylactic oxytocic agents?

A. 30%

B. 40%

C. 50%

D. 60%

E. 80%

217 A 33-year-old multiparous woman has been taking therapeutic low molecular weight heparin (LMWH) from 34 weeks gestation for confirmed pulmonary embolism. She has an uncomplicated spontaneous normal vaginal delivery at 38 weeks gestation.

What is the most appropriate postnatal management?

A. Continue therapeutic LMWH for 14 days postnatally

B. Continue therapeutic LMWH for a total of 3 months from the time of commencement of treatment

C. Switch to oral anticoagulant 24 hours after delivery

D. Switch to prophylactic LMWH and continue for 6 weeks post-natally

E. Switch to prophylactic LMWH and continue for a total of 3 months from time of commencement of treatment

218 A 37-year-old primigravida, 102 kg, and a BMI of 40 kg/m^2 is seen in the antenatal clinic for booking. She has conceived following a long period of subfertility through assisted conception. Ultrasound scan had confirmed a di-chorionic, di-amniotic twin pregnancy of 11+ 5 days gestation. Prophylactic LMWH had been given throughout pregnancy. A category 3 caesarean section had been performed at 37 weeks.

What is recommended as the best practice with regard to reducing maternal risk of VTE in the puerperium?

A. LMWH 20 mg per day for 6 weeks postnatally

B. LMWH 60 mg per day for 7 days postnatally

C. Prophylactic LMWH 60 mg per day for 6 weeks postnatally

D. TED stockings, mobilisation and hydration

E. Therapeutic LMWH for 7 days postnatally

219 A 25-year-old woman goes into spontaneous labour at term. She has an undiagnosed Chlamydia infection. What is the chance that she will develop a puerperal infection if she delivers vaginally?

A. 5%

B. 10%

C. 14%

D. 34%

E. 44%

220 Chlamydia testing should be performed in women with lower genital tract symptoms and intrapartum or postpartum fever, and in mothers of infants with ophthalmia neonatorum.

When should the test of cure be done after initial treatment in pregnancy?

A. 1–2 weeks after completion of treatment

B. 3–4weeks after completion of treatment

C. 5–6 weeks after completion of treatment

D. 7–8 weeks after completion of treatment

E. 9–10 weeks after completion of treatment

221 In a breastfeeding population, what is the risk of mother to child transmission of HIV due to breastfeeding?

A. 0–4%

B. 5–14%

C. 24–44%

D. 45–64%

E. 66–85%

222 What proportion of cases of neonatal Herpes simplex infection are due to HSV-2?

A. 10%

B. 20%

C. 30%

D. 40%

E. 50%

223 A woman with confirmed obstetric cholestatis has a normal vaginal delivery.

How long after delivery should repeat liver function tests be performed?

A. 48 hours

B. 5 days

C. 7 days

D. 10 days

E. 6 weeks

224 A woman in the second postpartum week presents with confusion, bewilderment, delusions and hallucinations. She feels hopeless and care of the baby has been affected.
What is the most likely diagnosis?
A. Baby blues
B. Postpartum psychosis
C. Severe pre-eclampsia
D. Severe sepsis
E. Substance abuse

225 Mental disorders during pregnancy and the postnatal period can have serious consequences on the health of the mother and her baby. It is vital that these women be managed by the appropriate health-care professionals.
Which health-care professional(s) should care for pregnant women with a history of postpartum psychosis?
A. Community mental health team
B. Community midwife
C. General obstetrician
D. General practitioner
E. Specialised perinatal mental health service

226 Postpartum psychosis is a psychiatric emergency usually needing admission.
What is the incidence of postpartum psychosis in the general population?
A. 1 in 100 deliveries
B. 1 in 1000 deliveries
C. 1 in 10,000 deliveries
D. 1 in 100,000 deliveries
E. 1 in 1,000,000 deliveries

227 A woman in the first postpartum week presents with mood swings ranging from elation to sadness, irritability, anxiety and decreased concentration. Care of the baby is not impaired and the woman does not feel suicidal.
What is the most likely diagnosis?
A. Baby blues
B. Postpartum psychosis
C. Severe pre-eclampsia
D. Severe sepsis
E. Substance abuse

228 At a woman's first contact with primary care or her booking visit and during the early postnatal period efforts should be made to ask about the woman's mental health and well-being using the 2 item GAD2 Scale:

What is the GAD-2 scale used for?

A. Identification of anxiety

B. Identification of bipolar disorder

C. Identification of depression

D. Risk of developing mania in pregnancy

E. Risk of puerperal psychosis

229 A woman with a history of severe depression presents with mild depression in pregnancy or the postnatal period.

What is the best plan of care?

A. Admit to mother and baby unit for further management

B. Commence pharmacotherapy

C. Consider ECT (Electro-convulsive therapy)

D. Offer CBT(Cognitive behaviour therapy)

E. Reassure and wait and watch

230 All health-care professionals providing assessment and interventions for mental health problems in pregnancy and the postnatal period should understand the variations in their presentation and course.

Along with this there should be knowledge of how these variations affect treatment, and the context in which they are assessed and treated (e.g., maternity services, health visiting and mental health services).

When a woman with a known or suspected mental health problem is referred in postnatal period within what time frame should assessment for treatment be initiated?

A. 2 weeks

B. 4 weeks

C. 6 weeks

D. 8 weeks

E. 10 weeks

Module 13

Gynaecological Problems

231 Following a spontaneous miscarriage at 8/40 gestation, a woman is referred to the gynaecology clinic with persistent irregular vaginal bleeding.

What initial investigation should be performed?

A. Endocervical swab to screen for chlamydia and gonorrhoea

B. Endometrial biopsy

C. Pelvic ultrasound scan

D. Serum βHCG level

E. Urinary pregnancy test

232 A 30-year-old woman attends the gynaecology clinic with discomfort in the left iliac fossa and clinical examination suggests a pelvic mass.

An ultrasound scan is arranged, which demonstrates a simple cyst in the left ovary with a diameter of 45 mm. The right ovary and uterus appear normal.

What other investigation is required?

A. Alfa-feto protein

B. CA-125

C. β-HCG

D. Lactate dehydrogenase

E. No investigation required

Part 2 MRCOG: Single Best Answer Questions, First Edition.
Andrew Sizer, Chandrika Balachandar, Nibedan Biswas, Richard Foon,
Anthony Griffiths, Sheena Hodgett, Banchhita Sahu and Martyn Underwood.
© 2016 John Wiley & Sons, Ltd. Published 2016 by John Wiley & Sons, Ltd.

233 A 40-year-old woman with BMI 32 kg/m² is referred to the gynae-cology clinic with secondary Amenorrhoea. She has two children and her partner had a vasectomy 5 years ago.

An ultrasound scan is performed, which shows a normal uterus with endometrial thickness 6 mm.

Both ovaries have a typical polycystic appearance.

What would be the recommended management?

A. Endometrial biopsy

B. Induction of 3-monthly withdrawal bleeds with progestagens

C. Metformin twice daily

D. Ovulation induction with clomiphene citrate

E. Reassure and discharge

234 A 55-year-old woman attends the gynaecology clinic. She is suffer-ing with terrible menopausal symptoms and cannot sleep because of the frequency of hot flushes.

She is requesting hormone replacement therapy (HRT) for symp-tom relief. She is currently healthy but has a history of a deep venous thrombosis in her calf following a fractured femur as a result of an accident 10 years ago.

Her last menstrual period was 2 years ago and her uterus is intact. What would you recommend?

A. All HRT is contraindicated in this situation

B. Oestrogen and testosterone implants

C. Oral continuous combined HRT

D. Raloxifene

E. Transdermal continuous combined HRT

235 A woman opts to take oral continuous combined HRT for 5 years after the menopause.

In which year of HRT use will her risk of venous thromboembolism (VTE) be greatest?

A. 1st year

B. 2nd year

C. 3rd year

D. 4th year

E. 5th year

236 What is the karyotype of a woman with Mayer–Rokitansky–Kuster–Hauser (MRKH) syndrome (mullerian agenesis)?

A. 45 XO

B. 46 XX

C. 46 XY

D. 47 XXX

E. 47 XXY

237 A 20-year-old girl attends the Gynaecology clinic with her mother. She presents with primary amenorrhoea.

On examination she is tall with a BMI of 19 kg/m². She has normal breast development, but a short blind-ending vagina. There is no axillary or pubic hair.

What is the most likely diagnosis?

A. Complete androgen insensitivity syndrome

B. Klinefelter syndrome

C. Mullerian agenesis

D. Swyer syndrome

E. Turners syndrome

238 A 48-year-old woman attends the gynaecology clinic complaining of heavy menstrual bleeding (HMB) and occasional intermenstrual bleeding.

Her haemoglobin level is 112 g/l.

An ultrasound scan demonstrated no obvious abnormality.

What other investigation is required?

A. Coagulation screen

B. Diagnostic hysteroscopy

C. Endometrial biopsy

D. MRI scan of pelvis

E. Serum FSH level

239 A 42-year-old woman with oligomenorrhoea and hirsutism presents to the gynaecology clinic. She recently had a prolonged episode of vaginal bleeding, but an ultrasound scan and endometrial biopsy performed in primary care both reported normal results. She is obese with a BMI of 40 kg/m². She has mild hypertension but does not require antihypertensive therapy. She has no other medical problems.

Her father suffered from Type 2 Diabetes mellitus.

What further investigation is required?

A. LH:FSH ratio

B. MRI scan of pelvis

C. Oral glucose tolerance test

D. Pregnancy test

E. Serum cholesterol

240 A 35-year-old woman attends the gynaecology clinic complaining of worsening HMB.
Investigations have been performed in primary care. Her haemoglobin level is 123 g/l and a pelvic ultrasound scan showed no obvious abnormality.
What is the most appropriate first-line pharmacological treatment?
A. Combined oral contraceptive pill
B. Cyclical Norethisterone
C. Depo Medroxyprogesterone acetate
D. Levonorgestrel-containing intrauterine system
E. Tranexamic acid

241 What percentage of women experience severe premenstrual symptoms?
A. 1%
B. 5%
C. 10%
D. 15%
E. 20%

242 The aetiology of premenstrual syndrome (PMS) remains unclear but appears to be related to the effect of cyclical ovarian activity on neurotransmitters.
Which neurotransmitters are considered to have a key role?
A. Adrenaline and Dopamine
B. Adrenaline and Noradrenaline
C. Gamma-aminobutyric acid (GABA) and Noradrenaline
D. Gamma-aminobutyric acid (GABA) and Serotonin
E. Serotonin and Dopamine

243 A 70-year-old woman undergoes a dual-energy X-ray absorptiometry (DXA) scan to assess her bone mineral density.
What T score is diagnostic of osteoporosis?
A. +2.5
B. +1.0
C. −1.0
D. −2.5
E. −5.0

244 What is the mode of action of bisphosphonates?
A. Calcitonin antagonist
B. Decreased bone resorption
C. Increased bone formation
D. Inhibition of release of parathyroid hormone
E. Vitamin D agonist

245 What is the most common side effect of bisphosphonates?
  A. Diarrhoea and vomiting
  B. Flu-like illness
  C. Oesophageal irritation
  D. Osteonecrosis of the jaw
  E. Urinary frequency

246 Raloxifene is a selective oestrogen receptor modulator.
  What kind of action does this drug have on the endometrium, breast and bone?

	Endometrium	Tissue Bone	Breast
A.	agonist	agonist	agonist
B.	agonist	antagonist	antagonist
C.	antagonist	agonist	antagonist
D.	antagonist	antagonist	agonist
E.	antagonist	antagonist	antagonist

247 A 29-year-old woman presents with a constant ongoing pain in the pelvis.
  The pain does not occur exclusively with menstruation or intercourse and the woman is not pregnant.
  For what minimum duration should the pain occur before it is deemed chronic?
  A. 1 week
  B. 1 month
  C. 3 months
  D. 6 months
  E. 1 year

248 An 18-year-old girl presents with chronic lower abdominal pain.
  In what percentage of patients attending a gynaecology outpatient clinic with lower abdominal/pelvic pain would you expect to find irritable bowel syndrome (IBS)?
  A. 10%
  B. 25%
  C. 33%
  D. 50%
  E. 66%

249 A 24-year-old girl attends the gynaecology clinic with persistent pain over her Pfannenstiel scar that has not settled since her caesarean section of 6 months.

What is the incidence of nerve entrapment (defined as highly localised, sharp, stabbing or aching pain, exacerbated by particular movements and persisting beyond 5 weeks or occurring after a pain free interval) after one Pfannenstiel incision ?

A. 1.7%
B. 3.7%
C. 5.7%
D. 7.7%
E. 9.7%

250 A 22-year-old girl presents with lower abdominal pain, which is cyclical in nature.

Which modality is the only way to reliably diagnose peritoneal endometriosis?

A. Computerised Tomography Scan of the abdomen and pelvis
B. Laparoscopy
C. Magnetic Resonance Imaging of the abdomen and pelvis
D. Trans-abdominal ultrasound scan of the abdomen
E. Trans-vaginal ultrasound scan of the pelvis

251 An 18-year-old girl with pelvic pain presents to the gynaecology outpatient clinic.

An ultrasound scan is arranged, which demonstrates a normal pelvis. Hormonal treatment is discussed with the girl.

How long should she persist with this therapy before contemplating a laparoscopy?

A. 1–3 months
B. 3–6 months
C. 6–9 months
D. 9–12 months
E. 1 year

252 What proportion of the female adult population will complain of chronic pelvic pain?

A. 1 in 2
B. 1 in 4
C. 1 in 6
D. 1 in 10
E. 1 in 20

253 A 19 year old has been seen in the gynaecology clinic with abdominal pain, which improves with defecation. It is associated with change in frequency of stool and change in form, for at least 3 days per month in the past 3 months.

What are the criteria used to define IBS?

A. Amsterdam criteria

B. Milan II criteria

C. Rome III criteria

D. Vienna II criteria

E. Zurich criteria

254 A 21 year old presents to the gynaecology outpatient clinic with pelvic pain. The general practitioner referral suggests possible endometriosis.

What is the estimated prevalence of endometriosis in women of reproductive age?

A. <1%

B. 2–10%

C. 10–20%

D. 25%

E. 50%

255 A 15-year-old girl is seen in the paediatric gynaecology clinic due to persistent vaginal discharge.

Examination reveals the following:

Partial removal of the clitoris and the prepuce is noted. The hymen is intact.

The possibility of female genital mutilation (FGM) is raised.

What type of FGM is this?

A. Type I

B. Type II

C. Type III

D. Type IV

E. It is not classed as FGM

256 A 21 year old who complains of superficial dyspareunia is seen in the gynaecology clinic. She has just started her first ever sexual relationship.

On examination, the following features are noted:

Normal vulva and vagina. Clitoris is intact. A piercing is noted in the right labium minorum.

What type of FGM is this?

A. Type I

B. Type II

C. Type III

D. Type IV

E. It is not classed as FGM

257 A 33-year-old woman is newly arrived in the United Kingdom from Africa and is complaining of dyspareunia.

How many women undergo FGM each year according to WHO estimates?

A. 500,000

B. 1 million

C. 2 million

D. 5 million

E. 10 million

258 A 24 year old has been seen in the antenatal clinic and is known to have undergone FGM. The lead midwife and health visitor are aware that any female offspring will be at risk of undergoing FGM. What is the estimated number of children in the United Kingdom that are considered to be at risk of this each year?

A. 500

B. 1000

C. 5000

D. 10,000

E. 20,000

259 A 13 year old attends the Accident & Emergency department with bleeding, pain and urinary retention following a recent FGM.

Which vaccine would you advise the patient to receive?

A. Hepatitis A

B. Hepatitis B

C. Hepatitis C

D. Tetanus toxoid

E. Varicella Zoster

260 What is the most common cause of central precocious puberty (CPP) in girls?

A. Craniopharyngioma

B. Hydrocephalus

C. Hypothalamic hamartoma

D. Idiopathic

E. McCune–Albright syndrome

261 A 47-year-old Para 3 who has had three previous vaginal deliveries presents with a history of HMB that has not responded to medical treatment or the levonorgestrel-containing intrauterine system (LNG-IUS). The patient was offered endometrial ablation but declined.

On examination, the uterus is bulky, no masses palpable in the adnexa and the cervix descends to about 2 cm above the hymenal ring. An ultrasound confirms the physical examination findings.

What is the most appropriate treatment option?

A. A combination of endometrial resection and levonorgestrel releasing-IUS

B. Laparoscopic vaginal assisted hysterectomy as it enables the surgeon to assess the pelvic organs

C. Subtotal hysterectomy as it avoids possible bladder injury and has a lower incidence of sexual dysfunction

D. Total abdominal hysterectomy as there is a lower risk of bladder injury than a vaginal hysterectomy

E. Vaginal hysterectomy

262 An asymptomatic postmenopausal woman is diagnosed with a simple unilateral unilocular cyst with a diameter of 4.5 cm. Her serum CA125 is 10 iu/l.

What is the most appropriate first line of management?

A. Discharge to GP

B. Follow up with ultrasound in 4 months time

C. Laparoscopic Bilateral salpingo-oophorectomy

D. Laparoscopic Unilateral salpingo-oophorectomy

E. Total abdominal hysterectomy with Bilateral salpingo-oophorectomy

263 The prevalence of ovarian cysts in premenopausal woman is higher than that in postmenopausal women; 35% versus 17% respectively.

A premenopausal woman presents with an asymptomatic 4.5 cm simple cyst in the left ovary with a serum CA125 of 18 iu/l.

What would be the recommended management plan?

A. Aspiration of the cyst under ultrasound guidance
B. Aspiration of the cyst under direct laparoscopic view
C. Hysterectomy in addition to bilateral salpingo-oophorectomy
D. Laparoscopic left salpingo-oophorectomy
E. Reassure and manage conservatively

264 A 40-year-old woman complains of burning and stinging in the vulva. There is no clinically identifiable neurological condition and there are no relevant visible findings.

What is the most likely clinical diagnosis?

A. Atrophic vaginitis
B. Herpes neuralgia
C. Immunobullous disorder
D. Lichen planus
E. Vulvodynia

265 A women diagnosed with localised unprovoked vulvodynia has had no relief from her symptoms despite practising good vulval care and using topical treatments which included lidocaine ointment and gabapentin.

What is the next line of management?

A. Anticonvulsant therapy
B. Laser ablation of Vulva
C. Modified vestibulectomy
D. Transcutaneous electrical nerve stimulation
E. Tricyclic antidepressant drugs

266 Community-based surveys indicate that about one-fifth of women have significant vulval symptoms.

Symptoms and signs of vulval skin disorders are common and include pruritus, pain and changes in skin colour and texture.

What is the most common vulval disorder seen in a hospital setting?

A. Dermatitis
B. Lichen planus
C. Lichen sclerosus
D. Lichen simplex
E. Vulval Candidiasis

267 Lichen sclerosus accounts for at least 25% of the women seen in dedicated vulval clinics, with estimates of incidence quoted as 1 in 300 to 1 in 1000 of all patients referred to dermatology departments.

What is the pathognomonic histologic feature of lichen sclerosus?

A. Acanthosis, hyperkeratosis and upper dermal fibrosis
B. Hyalisation of upper dermis
C. Plasma cells in a dense inflammatory infilterate
D. Squamous hyperplasia and a chronic perivascular inflammation
E. Thinning and effacement of the squamous epithelium with chronic upper dermal inflammation

268 A 60-year-old woman presents with vulval itching with no relief with scratching.

On examination the skin appears fragile, with well demarcated white plaques. There is no involvement of the vagina or the oral mucosa.

What is the most likely diagnosis?

A. Lichen Planus
B. Lichen sclerosus
C. Lichen simplex chronicus
D. Vulval dermatitis
E. Vulval psoriasis

269 A woman with biopsy-proven lichen sclerosus is not responding to topical ultra-potent steroids.

What is the second line of treatment?

A. CO_2 Laser vaporisation
B. Local surgical excision
C. Topical emollient
D. Topical imiquimod cream
E. Topical Tacrolimus

270 A 25-year-old smoker is diagnosed to have mild dyskariosis in her index smear at the GP surgery. The smear is HPV negative.

What is the ideal management?

A. Reassure and discharge for repeat smear in 3 years
B. Referral to colposcopy for review
C. Repeat smear in 12 months and if still has mild dyskariosis refer for colposcopy
D. Repeat smear in 3 months and if still has mild dyskariosis refer for colposcopy
E. Repeat smear in 6 months and if still has mild dyskariosis refer for colposcopy

271 A 40-year-old woman attends for a consultation in primary care complaining of HMB. She is otherwise fit and well and examination is unremarkable.

What investigation should be undertaken?

A. Coagulation screen
B. Endometrial biopsy
C. Full blood count
D. Pelvic ultrasound scan
E. Serum ferritin

272 Following referral to secondary care for HMB, a 38-year old woman undergoes pelvic examination, which confirms that the uterus is palpable abdominally.

What is the first line diagnostic test to identify structural abnormalities in this situation?

A. CT scan
B. Hysteroscopy
C. MRI scan
D. Pelvic ultrasound scan
E. Saline infusion sonography

273 A 39-year-old woman presents to the gynaecology clinic with HMB and dysmenorrhoea. She is otherwise fit and well.

Pelvic examination is unremarkable.

She is not keen on hormonal methods of treatment.

What treatment would you initially recommend?

A. Danazol
B. Etamsylate
C. Mefenemic acid
D. Norethisterone
E. Tranexamic acid

274 A 38-year-old woman is seen in the gynaecology clinic. She presented with HMB.

History and examination are unremarkable and she is commenced on tranexamic acid, to be taken during menstruation only.

Should this treatment ultimately prove to be ineffective, for how many cycles should she have tried it to come to this conclusion?

A. 3 cycles
B. 6 cycles
C. 9 cycles
D. 12 cycles
E. 18 cycles

275 During investigation for HMB, a 42-year-old woman is found to have a 3 cm submucus fibroid.

She is otherwise fit and well. Her husband has had a vasectomy. She does not wish to try pharmaceutical treatments.

What would you recommend?

A. Hysteroscopic resection of fibroid and endometrium

B. Novasure endometrial ablation

C. Open myomectomy

D. Total abdominal hysterectomy

E. Uterine artery embolization

276 A 55-year-old woman attends the general practitioner surgery with abdominal distension, low abdominal pain and urinary urgency.

Abdominal examination is unremarkable and urine dipstick is negative.

What investigation should be performed?

A. CT scan urinary tract

B. Full blood count

C. No investigation – reassure and discharge

D. Pelvic ultrasound scan

E. Serum CA125

277 What screening test should be offered to all sexually active women who present to the gynaecology clinic with chronic pelvic pain?

A. Endocervical swabs for Chlamydia and Gonorrhoea

B. Magnetic resonance imaging

C. Serum CA125

D. Serum C-reactive protein

E. Transvaginal ultrasound

278 After a year of 4-monthly follow-up, a healthy 75-year-old woman with a 5 cm simple unilocular ovarian cyst and a normal serum CA-125 level decides that she would prefer to have surgical treatment.

What treatment would you recommend?

A. Aspiration of the cyst

B. Laparoscopic bilateral oophorectomy

C. Laparoscopic ovarian cystectomy

D. Laparoscopic unilateral oophorectomy

E. Total abdominal hysterectomy and bilateral salpingo-oophorectomy

279 Following a diagnosis of anogenital lichen sclerosus, a 70-year-old woman returns to clinic as topical potent steroids have not been effective in controlling her symptoms.

The recommended second-line treatment is Tacrolimus.

Which cell type of the immune system has its response suppressed by this drug?

A. B lymphocytes
B. Macrophages
C. Natural killer cells
D. Plasma cells
E. T lymphocytes

280 Which progestagen has been shown to be effective in cases of PMS?

A. Desogestrel
B. Drospirenone
C. Levonorgestrel
D. Medroxyprogesterone acetate
E. Norethisterone

Module 14

Subfertility

281 A 28-year-old amenorrhoeic woman who wishes to become pregnant attends the fertility clinic complaining of galactorrhoea and mild visual disturbance. Her serum prolactin level was found to be elevated.

An MRI scan of the head is performed, which showed the presence of a macroprolactinoma, but without supracellar extension.

What is the most appropriate first line management?

A. Bromocriptine

B. Cabergoline

C. Quinagolide

D. Radiotherapy

E. Trans-sphenoidal surgical excision of the prolactinoma

282 In the female, which cell type secretes Anti-Mullerian hormone?

A. Granulosa cells

B. Leydig cells

C. Primary oocytes

D. Secondary Oocytes

E. Sertoli cells

283 A woman with tubal disease is advised to have IVF treatment to maximise her chances of pregnancy. On reading the information leaflet, she is very concerned about the risks of ovarian hyperstimulation syndrome.

What is the chance of developing severe ovarian hyperstimulation syndrome (OHSS) and requiring hospitalisation in women undergoing controlled ovarian hyperstimulation?

A. 0.1–0.2 %

B. 1–3%

C. 8–10%

D. 15–20%

E. 30–40%

Part 2 MRCOG: Single Best Answer Questions, First Edition.
Andrew Sizer, Chandrika Balachandar, Nibedan Biswas, Richard Foon, Anthony Griffiths, Sheena Hodgett, Banchhita Sahu and Martyn Underwood.
© 2016 John Wiley & Sons, Ltd. Published 2016 by John Wiley & Sons, Ltd.

284 What is the predominant cause of anovulatory infertility?
A. Hyperprolactinemia
B. Hypogonadotrophic hypogonadism
C. Obesity
D. Polycystic ovary syndrome
E. Premature ovarian failure

285 What is the first-line pharmacological treatment for anovulatory polycystic ovary syndrome?
A. Anastrozole
B. Clomifene
C. Letrozole
D. Recombinant FSH
E. Tamoxifen

286 A 32-year-old woman presents to the gynaecology clinic with galactorrhoea and secondary amenorrhoea. A serum prolactin level is measured and found to be elevated.
What is the main mechanism by which hyperprolactinemia causes secondary amenorrhoea?
A. Disruption of granulosa cell development
B. Induction of atrophic changes in the endometrium
C. Inhibition of follicle stimulating hormone (FSH) pulsatility
D. Inhibition of luteinsing hormone (LH) pulsatility
E. Inhibition of meiosis in the developing oocyte

287 Following an IVF treatment cycle where 15 oocytes were collected, a patient presents to the clinic with abdominal pain, nausea and vomiting.
An ultrasound scan is performed, which shows the ovaries to be enlarged with a mean diameter of 10cm. There is a small amount of ascites.
What is the diagnosis?
A. Critical OHSS
B. Mild OHSS
C. Moderate OHSS
D. Normal findings post oocyte-retrieval
E. Severe OHSS

288 What type of electrolyte disturbance is often seen in association with severe cases of OHSS ?
A. Hypercalcaemia
B. Hyperkalaemia
C. Hypernatraemia
D. Hypokalaemia
E. Hyponatraemia

289 A woman with a severe cases of OHSS initially presented with tense ascites, oliguria and a haematocrit of 46%.

She was treated with appropriate fluid replacement and the haematocrit is now in the normal range.

However, she remains markedly oliguric.

What is the appropriate management?

A. Bendroflumethazide orally
B. Furosemide IV
C. Haemodialysis
D. Ongoing intravenous fluids at a rate of 5–6 l/24 hours
E. Paracentesis

290 What is the recommended test for the biochemical detection of hyperandrogenism?

A. 17-hydroxy progesterone
B. Free androgen index
C. Free testosterone
D. Sex-hormone binding globulin
E. Total testosterone

291 What proportion of women with polycystic ovarian syndrome are overweight/obese?

A. 10–20%
B. 40–50%
C. 60–70%
D. 80–85%
E. 95–100%

292 What is the mechanism of action of Metformin?

A. Enhances insulin sensitivity at the cellular level
B. Increases renal glucose reabsorption
C. Inhibits insulin release
D. Promotes hepatic glycogenolysis
E. Promotes hepatic gluconeogenesis

293 What is the estimated prevalence of endometriosis in infertile women?

A. 10%
B. 20%
C. 30%
D. 40%
E. 50%

294 During fertility investigations, a woman is found to be susceptible to Rubella and is offered vaccination.

How long should she use contraception before trying to conceive again?

A. 1 month

B. 3 months

C. 6 months

D. 12 months

E. Can try and conceive immediately

295 Following fertility investigations, a man is found to have idiopathic oligozoospermia.

He enquires if there is any treatment he can take to improve his sperm count.

What would you recommend?

A. Androstenedione

B. Clomiphene citrate

C. Letrozole

D. No treatment is of proven benefit

E. Recombinant FSH

296 Following a full set of investigations in the fertility clinic, a couple are diagnosed as having unexplained infertility since all the tests have been reported as normal.

The couple have been trying to conceive for 3 years.

What treatment would be recommended?

A. Conservative management

B. Ovulation induction with Clomiphene citrate

C. Ovulation induction with Letrozole

D. Intracytoplasmic sperm injection (ICSI)

E. In vitro fertilisation (IVF)

297 Prior to a frozen embryo transfer, a woman takes a course of oestradiol valerate to induce endometrial proliferation.

She attends for an ultrasound scan after 10 days to measure the endometrial thickness.

What endometrial thickness should have been achieved in order for the embryo transfer to proceed?

A. 1mm

B. 2mm

C. 3mm

D. 4mm

E. 5mm

298 Which form of contraception is most strongly associated with a delay in return of fertility?
A. Copper-containing intrauterine device
B. Depo medroxyprogesterone acetate
C. Etonorgestrel-containing subdermal implant
D. Levonorgestrel containing intrauterine system
E. Progestogen-only pill

299 Fertility declines with age.
What percentage of women aged 35 will take longer than a year to conceive with regular intercourse?
A. 5%
B. 15%
C. 30%
D. 45%
E. 60%

300 According to the current WHO criteria, what is the reference limit for the total number of spermatozoa in an ejaculate?
A. 4×10^6
B. 15×10^6
C. 32×10^6
D. 39×10^6
E. 58×10^6

Module 15

Sexual and Reproductive Health

301 In the United Kingdom, which synthetic oestrogen is contained in most combined oral contraceptive (COC) pills?
- **A.** Cyproterone acetate
- **B.** Drospirenone
- **C.** Ethinylestradiol
- **D.** Oestradiol valerate
- **E.** Mestranol

302 What is the primary mode of action of the progestogen-only injectable method of contraception (Depo Provera)?
- **A.** Endometrial atrophy
- **B.** Inhibition of ovulation
- **C.** Prevention of fertilisation
- **D.** Prevention of implantation
- **E.** Thickening of cervical mucus

303 What is the most efficacious form of long-acting reversible contraception?
- **A.** COC pill
- **B.** Copper intrauterine device
- **C.** Depo medroxyprogesterone acetate
- **D.** Etonorgestrel-containing subdermal implant
- **E.** Levonorgestrel-containing intrauterine system

304 Which form of progestogen-only contraception is most strongly associated with loss of bone mineral density?
- **A.** Depo medroxyprogesterone acetate
- **B.** Depo norethisterone enantate
- **C.** Etonorgestrel-containing subdermal implant
- **D.** Levonorgestrel-containing intrauterine system
- **E.** Progestogen-only pill

Part 2 MRCOG: Single Best Answer Questions, First Edition.
Andrew Sizer, Chandrika Balachandar, Nibedan Biswas, Richard Foon, Anthony Griffiths, Sheena Hodgett, Banchhita Sahu and Martyn Underwood.
© 2016 John Wiley & Sons, Ltd. Published 2016 by John Wiley & Sons, Ltd.

305 Which form of long-acting reversible contraception is least suitable for use in adolescents?
  A. COC pill
  B. Copper intrauterine device
  C. Depo medroxyprogesterone acetate
  D. Etonorgestrel-containing subdermal implant
  E. Levonorgestrel-containing intrauterine system

306 Which two drugs are the only selective progesterone receptor modulators (SPRMs) licensed for use in the United Kingdom?
  A. Medroxyprogesterone acetate and Ulipristal acetate
  B. Mifepristone and Misoprostol
  C. Mifepristone and Tibolone
  D. Mifepristone and Ulipristal acetate
  E. Tibolone and Drospirenone

307 What is the background rate of venous thromboembolism (VTE) in women of reproductive age?
  A. 10/100,000/year
  B. 20/100,000/year
  C. 50/100,000/year
  D. 100/100,000/year
  E. 200/100,000/year

308 A woman switches from a COC pill containing ethinyloestradiol and levonorgestrel to a different pill containing ethinyloestradiol and desogestrel. The dose of ethinyloestradiol is the same in both preparations.
  Approximately, by how many times will she have increased her risk of VTE?
  A. 2
  B. 5
  C. 10
  D. 15
  E. 20

309 What is the primary mode of action by which the COC pill exerts its contraceptive effect?
  A. Endometrial atrophy
  B. Inhibition of ovulation
  C. Sperm immobilisation
  D. Suppression of meiosis
  E. Thickening of cervical mucus

310 What percentage of women with gonorrhoea are coinfected with chlamydia?
A. 10%
B. 20%
C. 30%
D. 40%
E. 50%

311 Gonorrhoea infection in pregnancy increases the risk of preterm rupture of membranes, preterm birth and low birth weight.
What percentage of exposed babies would develop Ophthalmia neonatorum?
A. 50%
B. 60%
C. 70%
D. 80%
E. 90%

312 Trichomonas vaginalis infection in pregnancy is associated with preterm birth and low birth weight.
What percentage of infected women are asymptomatic?
A. 10–50%
B. 50–60%
C. 60–70%
D. 70–80%
E. 80–90%

313 Vertical transmission of human papilloma virus (HPV) can cause genital and laryngeal warts and recurrent respiratory papillomatosis in infants.
What is the risk of vertical transmission?
A. 1 in 1000 cases
B. 1 in 500 cases
C. 1 in 150 cases
D. 1 in 80 cases
E. 1 in 50 cases

314 Most cases of syphilis in pregnancy are detected through antenatal screening. The management should involve a multidisciplinary team of obstetricians, genitourinary physicians and neonatologists. Penicillin is the treatment of choice.

What percentage of cases develop the Jarisch–Herxheimer reaction during treatment of syphilis in pregnancy?

A. 5%
B. 25%
C. 45%
D. 65%
E. 85%

315 Vasectomy failure rate is quoted as approximately 1 in 2000 (0.05%) after clearance has been given.

By how many months postprocedure should the vasectomy be considered a failure if motile sperm are still observed in a fresh semen sample?

A. 3 months
B. 4 months
C. 5 months
D. 6 months
E. 7 months

316 Ulipristal acetate (UPA) may itself reduce the efficacy of other hormonal contraception.

When emergency contraception is administered because of a missed combined oral contraceptive pill (CHC) the CHC should be continued.

For how many days should additional contraception be advised?

A. 0 days
B. 7 days
C. 14 days
D. 21 days
E. 28 days

317 Besides providing reliable contraception, COC offers a variety of noncontraceptive health benefits.

What percentage of women of reproductive age use COCs for contraception in the United Kingdom?

A. 7%
B. 17%
C. 27%
D. 37%
E. 47%

318 Reproductive coercion is defined as the attempt by men to control their female partners' pregnancies and pregnancy outcomes.
What is the reported percentage of incidence of birth control sabotage by male partners?
A. 25%
B. 35%
C. 45%
D. 55%
E. 65%

319 More and more women are leaving childbearing to a later age.
What is the most common reason given by women for making this choice?
A. Availability of reliable contraceptives
B. Career concerns
C. Financial reasons
D. Finding a suitable partner
E. Other causes

320 As a post coital contraception, the primary mechanism of action of Ulipristal acetate is inhibition of ovulation.
What is the conception rate when Ulipristal acetate is taken within 120 hours of unprotected sexual intercourse?
A. 1.3%
B. 2.3%
C. 3.3%
D. 4.3%
E. 5.3%

Module 16

Early Pregnancy Problems

321 A woman attends her first ultrasound scan in pregnancy. What is the maximum crown rump length (CRL) that is accurate for dating before you measure gestational age by head circumference (HC)

    A. 14 mm

    B. 24 mm

    C. 44 mm

    D. 84 mm

    E. 94 mm

322 At what gestational age is chorionic villus sampling (CVS) usually performed?

    A. $8–10^{+0}$ gestation

    B. $8–13^{+6}$ gestation

    C. $10–11^{+0}$ gestation

    D. $11–13^{+6}$ gestation

    E. $12–14^{+6}$ gestation

323 A woman is currently being treated for acne with oral retinoids and finds herself pregnant in the first trimester. What is her chance of miscarrying?

    A. 5%

    B. 10–15%

    C. 20–40%

    D. 30–50%

    E. 80–90%

Part 2 MRCOG: Single Best Answer Questions, First Edition.
Andrew Sizer, Chandrika Balachandar, Nibedan Biswas, Richard Foon,
Anthony Griffiths, Sheena Hodgett, Banchhita Sahu and Martyn Underwood.
© 2016 John Wiley & Sons, Ltd. Published 2016 by John Wiley & Sons, Ltd.

324 A woman presents at 8 weeks gestation in her first pregnancy with severe nausea and vomiting of pregnancy (NVP). Her thyroid function test (TFT) results are as follows:

TSH: 0.1 mU/l

FT4: 20 pmol/l

What is the most appropriate management plan?
- **A.** Commence carbimazole and check TSH receptor antibodies
- **B.** Commence propylthiouracil (PTU) and repeat TFT in 6 weeks
- **C.** Supportive treatment for NVP and check TSH receptor antibodies
- **D.** Supportive treatment for NVP and repeat TFT in 6 weeks
- **E.** Supportive treatment for NVP only

325 A 30-year-old woman visits her GP at 8 weeks gestation in her second pregnancy with mild symptoms of nausea and vomiting of pregnancy (NVP). She had severe NVP in her first pregnancy requiring hospital admission and is concerned that her symptoms will worsen.

What is the most appropriate advice from her GP?
- **A.** Admission to hospital for assessment and treatment
- **B.** Outpatient hospital attendance for intravenous rehydration
- **C.** Reassurance that severe NVP is unlikely to recur
- **D.** Treatment with cyclizine if symptoms worsen
- **E.** Treatment with ondansetron if symptoms worsen

326 What percentage of pregnant women with hyperemesis gravidarum in early pregnancy experience transient hyperthyroidism?
- **A.** 20%
- **B.** 30%
- **C.** 40%
- **D.** 50%
- **E.** 60%

327 A 26-year-old patient presents with left iliac fossa pain and has a 6 week period of amenorrhoea. The patient is clinically stable. An ultrasound confirms the presence of a left-sided ectopic pregnancy. There is a 2x2x2 cm pool of free fluid in the pouch of Douglas and the serum βHCG level is 3500 IU/l.

What is the recommended management?
- **A.** Left Laparoscopic salpingectomy, if the contralateral tube is healthy
- **B.** Left Laparoscopic Salpingotomy
- **C.** Left Salpingectomy via a laparotomy
- **D.** Methotrexate
- **E.** Repeat the βHCG levels and manage accordingly

328 A woman has undergone surgical management of miscarriage and a partial molar pregnancy has been confirmed. Referral to a specialist centre is advised.

Where are the three specialist referral centres in the United Kingdom?

A. Aberdeen, Birmingham, London

B. Cardiff, Edinburgh, London

C. Dundee, London, Sheffield

D. Edinburgh, London, Sheffield

E. Glasgow, London, Sheffield

329 A woman has undergone surgical management of miscarriage and the histology confirms Gestational Trophoblastic Disease (GTD).

What is the expected incidence of GTD in the United Kingdom?

A. 1 in 214 live births

B. 1 in 714 live births

C. 1 in 1254 live births

D. 1 in 2544 live births

E. 1 in 7140 live births

330 A woman has been diagnosed with high-risk gestational trophoblastic neoplasia (GTN) and is about to receive multiagent chemotherapy.

What is the expected cure rate?

A. 65%

B. 75%

C. 85%

D. 95%

E. 100%

331 A woman has attended the gynaecology clinic to discuss a diagnosis of a molar pregnancy.

What is the definitive method of diagnosis?

A. Clinical assessment

B. Histologic analysis of tissue

C. Serum βHCG levels

D. Ultrasound

E. Urine βHCG levels

332 A woman underwent medical management of miscarriage but no specimen was sent for histological analysis.

What would be the advice to the patient following this procedure?

A. Do nothing

B. If your period does not return within 6 weeks do a home pregnancy test

C. Perform a home pregnancy test in 1 week

D. Perform a home pregnancy test in 3 weeks

E. Perform a home pregnancy test in 5 weeks

333 During a routine surgical evacuation of miscarriage when should oxytocic agents be used?

A. Always

B. If blood loss exceeds 50 ml

C. If blood loss exceeds 150 ml

D. If blood loss exceeds 250 ml

E. If life-threatening bleeding is encountered

334 A woman has had surgical management of miscarriage and a molar pregnancy has been confirmed.

Which immunohistochemistry marker is useful for distinguishing between partial and complete molar pregnancies?

A. P16

B. P53

C. P57

D. P87

E. P96

335 A woman has had an ultrasound scan and the possibility of a molar pregnancy with a co-existing twin has been raised by the sonographer.

The woman has been referred to a regional fetal medicine centre for further investigations.

What would be the most appropriate investigation?

A. Fetal blood sampling for βHCG levels of the suspected molar pregnancy

B. Karyotyping of the suspected molar pregnancy

C. Karyotyping of the mother

D. MRI scan

E. Serum βHCG levels

336 What percentage of partial molar pregnancies consist of tetraploid or mosaic conceptions?

A. 10%

B. 25%

C. 50%

D. 75%

E. 90%

337 A 25-year-old woman attends the Early Pregnancy Unit with vomiting and bleeding. An ultrasound scan is performed, which is strongly suggestive of a molar pregnancy.

What is the optimal method of uterine evacuation?

A. Medical evacuation with Methotrexate

B. Medical evacuation with Mifepristone and Misoprostol

C. Medical Evacuation with Oxytocin

D. Suction curettage

E. Total Hysterectomy

338 A 30-year-old woman attends the preconception counselling clinic. She has completed follow-up with the regional trophoblastic screening centre following a partial molar pregnancy.

She is keen to try and conceive again, but wishes to know the risk of a further molar pregnancy.

What would you tell her the risk is?

A. 1/10

B. 1/25

C. 1/50

D. 1/80

E. 1/200

339 A woman attends the early pregnancy unit having experienced her second successive miscarriage.

She has been researching miscarriage on the internet and has read that most miscarriages are due to genetic problems.

What percentage of first-trimester miscarriages are due to chromosomal abnormalities?

A. 50%

B. 60%

C. 70%

D. 80%

E. 90%

340 What is the age-related risk of miscarriage in women under 20 years of age?

A. 5%

B. 13%

C. 20%

D. 28%

E. 35%

341 A woman attends the miscarriage clinic having experienced her third consecutive first-trimester loss.

Which investigations should be undertaken?

	Investigation					
	Antiphos-pholipid antibodies	Karyo-typing of both parents	Pelvic ultra-sound scan	Thrombo-philia screen	Cyto-genetics of products of conception	Maternal peripheral natural killer cells	TORCH screen
A.	X	X		X		X	
B.	X		X	X	X		
C.	X	X				X	X
D.		X	X	X			X
E.	X		X		X		

342 Which B vitamin has been shown to be effective in the reduction of nausea and vomiting of pregnancy (NVP)?

A. Cobalamin

B. Folic acid

C. Pyridoxine

D. Riboflavin

E. Thiamine

343 A 30-year-old woman attends the early pregnancy unit with a positive pregnancy test and some lower abdominal pain. Her last menstrual period was approximately 8 weeks ago, but her menstrual cycle is irregular.

A transvaginal ultrasound scan is organised, which demonstrates an intrauterine gestation sac with fetal pole and yolk sac, but no fetal heartbeat is identified. The crown-rump length (CRL) is 6mm. What is the correct course of action?

A. Inform the woman that she has a missed miscarriage and arrange surgical evacuation

B. Inform the woman that she has a missed miscarriage and arrange medical evacuation with misoprostol

C. Inform the woman that she has a missed miscarriage and arrange medical evacuation with mifepristone and misoprostol

D. Inform the woman that the pregnancy appears normal and no further intervention is required

E. Inform the woman that the viability of the pregnancy is uncertain and arrange for a further scan in 7–10 days

344 A woman who has had a left salpingectomy previously for ectopic pregnancy has now been diagnosed with an ectopic pregnancy in the right fallopian tube.

A laparoscopy is performed and the surgeon opts for a salpingotomy as the woman still wishes to become pregnant. What is the possibility that she will require further treatment (methotrexate or salpingectomy)?

A. 1%

B. 5%

C. 10%

D. 20%

E. 50%

345 A woman attends the early pregnancy unit and has a confirmed diagnosis of miscarriage. She is fit and well, and all observations are normal.

What is the recommended first line management?

A. Evacuation of retained products of conception

B. Expectant management for 7–14 days

C. Intramuscular Methotrexate

D. Oral Mifepristone

E. Vaginal Misoprostol

346 A woman who has blood group A Rh negative undergoes a laparo-scopic salpingectomy for a ruptured ectopic pregnancy.

What anti-D rhesus prophylaxis is required?

A. 250 IU anti-D

B. 500 IU anti-D

C. Two doses of 250 IU anti-D 48 hours apart

D. No prophylaxis required

E. Quantify the feto-maternal haemorrhage with a Kleihauer test to determine the correct dose of anti-D

347 A woman underwent a surgical evacuation of the uterus following a failed intrauterine pregnancy.

The products of conception were sent for histological analysis and a diagnosis of complete molar pregnancy was made.

The woman was referred to the regional trophoblastic disease centre for follow-up, and subsequently required treatment with single-agent chemotherapy.

She returns to clinic after completion of treatment as she wishes to conceive again.

How long should she wait?

A. 1 month

B. 3 months

C. 6 months

D. 12 months

E. 18 months

348 A woman attends for her first trimester dating scan at 12 weeks gestation and all appears well. Both fetal heart and fetal move-ments are seen.

What is the chance that she will miscarry before 24 weeks of gestation?

A. 0.1–0.2%

B. 0.5–0.6%

C. 1–2%

D. 5–6%

E. 10–15%

349 What investigation is indicated for women following a second-trimester miscarriage, which is not indicated in recurrent first-trimester loss?

A. Anticardiolipin antibodies

B. Karyotyping of products of conception

C. Lupus anticoagulant

D. Pelvic ultrasound scan

E. Thrombophilia screen

350 A healthy 30-year-old woman with recurrent first-trimester miscarriage attends the clinic for investigation and all tests recommended in the RCOG guideline are reported as normal.

The woman is a member of an internet support group for miscarriage and has heard from other members that there may be other adjunctive treatments that can be used.

What treatment would you recommend?

A. HCG supplementation

B. Immunoglobulin intravenously

C. No adjunctive treatment of proven benefit in this situation

D. Paternal white cell transfusion

E. Progesterone supplementation

Module 17

Gynaecological Oncology

351 Administration of tamoxifen is a cornerstone in the treatment of breast cancer, but it has a weak estrogenic effect on the endometrium.

A woman who is taking Tamoxifen presents with post-menopausal bleeding (PMB).

What is her risk of developing endometrial cancer when compared to the general population?

A. No increased risk
B. 1–2 times
C. 3–6 times
D. 8–10 times
E. 15–20 times

352 PMB is defined as uterine bleeding occurring after at least one year of amenorrhoea. The main purpose of investigating a woman with PMB is to rule out endometrial cancer.

What is the risk that a women presenting with PMB will have endometrial cancer?

A. 5–10%
B. 10–15%
C. 15–20%
D. 20–25%
E. 25–30%

Part 2 MRCOG: Single Best Answer Questions, First Edition.
Andrew Sizer, Chandrika Balachandar, Nibedan Biswas, Richard Foon, Anthony Griffiths, Sheena Hodgett, Banchhita Sahu and Martyn Underwood.

353 A 60-year-old woman presents with a first episode of PMB.
What is the most appropriate first line of investigation?
   A. Dilatation and Curettage to assess the endometrium
   B. Hysteroscopy to assess the endometrial cavity and obtain an endometrial sample
   C. Pipelle biopsy to obtain an endometrial sample
   D. Saline infusion sonography to measure the endometrial thickness
   E. Transvaginal sonography to assess the endometrial thickness

354 A 55-year-old woman presents with a first episode of PMB. A transvaginal ultrasound scan showed an endometrial thickness of 3.8 mm.
What is the most appropriate management plan?
   A. Book a repeat transvaginal scan in 6 months
   B. Book for an out-patient hysteroscopy to look at endometrial cavity and obtain endometrial sample
   C. Perform a dilatation and curettage
   D. Perform an endometrial sampling to rule out endometrial cancer
   E. Reassure, follow expectant management

355 A 60 year old undergoes hysterectomy and bilateral salpingo-oophorectomy for grade 1 endometrial cancer.
The final histology report confirms tumor invading the uterine serosa.
As per the new FIGO staging of endometrial cancer, what is the stage?
   A. Stage IC
   B. Stage IIC
   C. Stage IIIA
   D. Stage IIIB
   E. Stage IIIC

356 Ovarian cysts are common in postmenopausal women, although their prevalence is lower than in premenopausal women.
A 59-year-old woman is referred to the clinic with fullness in the lower abdomen and a serum CA125 level of 64iu/l.
What is the first line of investigation?
   A. Computed Tomography (CT) of abdomen and pelvis
   B. MRI of pelvis
   C. PET scan
   D. Transvaginal ultrasound scan of pelvis
   E. USS of pelvis with Doppler

357 It is recommended that 'risk of malignancy index' (RMI) should be used to triage post-menopausal women with an ovarian cyst to assess low, moderate or high risk of malignancy.

This is calculated as U (ultrasound score) X M (menopausal status) X CA125.

What is the RMI of a post-menopausal woman with a CA125 of 15, ultrasound showing 6 cm bilateral, multiloculated cyst?

A. 45
B. 90
C. 95
D. 130
E. 135

358 It is recommended that RMI should be used to triage post-menopausal women with ovarian cyst to assess low, moderate or high risk of malignancy.

This is calculated as U (ultrasound score) × M (menopausal status) × CA125.

What is the risk of ovarian cancer in a woman who has an RMI of 25–250 (moderate risk)?

A. 3%
B. 20%
C. 25%
D. 60%
E. 75%

359 Who should be responsible for the management of women with intermediate risk of malignancy (RMI of 25–250)?

A. General gynecologist in a cancer centre
B. General gynaecologist in a cancer unit
C. General gynaecologist in a district general hospital
D. Gynaecological oncologist in a cancer centre
E. Lead clinician in a cancer unit

360 Borderline ovarian tumors are a distinct pathological group of neoplasms typically seen in younger women. They are often diagnosed at an earlier stage resulting in excellent prognosis.

What is the histologic feature that differentiates borderline ovarian tumors from invasive ovarian cancers?

A. Absence of hyperchromasia
B. Absence of stromal invasion
C. Presence of extra ovarian invasive implants
D. Presence of mitotic figures
E. Presence of prominent nucleoli

361 A 49-year-old para 3 underwent laparoscopic left salpingo-oophorectomy for a complex left ovarian cyst. Histology shows a serous micro papillary borderline ovarian tumor with the presence of DNA aneuploidy.

What is the most appropriate management plan?

A. CT scan in 6 months time

B. Reassure and discharge

C. Right salpingo-oophorectomy

D. Total abdominal hysterectomy and right salpingo-oophorectomy

E. Total abdominal hysterectomy and right salpingo-oophorectomy, peritoneal washings, infracolic omentectomy and exploration of entire abdominal cavity

362 Borderline ovarian tumors are also known as tumors of low malignant potential. They constitute 10–15% of all epithelial ovarian neoplasms.

What is the 5-year survival rate of stage 1 borderline ovarian tumor?

A. 75–77%

B. 80–83%

C. 85–87%

D. 90–93%

E. 95–97%

363 The lifetime risk of ovarian cancer in the general population is 1.4%. However, women with hereditary ovarian cancer syndrome have significantly higher risks of developing ovarian cancer.

What is the risk of ovarian cancer in a woman who has a BRCA1 mutation carrier?

A. 15–25%

B. 25–35%

C. 35–45%

D. 45–55%

E. 55–65%

364 Lynch syndrome, also called hereditary nonpolyposis colorectal cancer (HNPCC) is associated with the development of multiple types of cancer.

What is the suggested management for reduction of risk of developing gynaecological cancers in a 35-year-old woman with HNPCC who has completed her family?

A. 6 monthly CA125 and transvaginal ultrasound

B. 12 monthly CA125 and transvaginal ultrasound

C. Hysterectomy and bilateral salpingo-oophorectomy

D. Laparoscopic bilateral salpingo-oophorectomy

E. Regular use of combined oral contraceptive pills

365 NICE recommends not to include systematic retroperitoneal lymphadenectomy as part of standard surgical treatment in women with suspected ovarian cancer whose disease appears to be confined to the ovaries (that is, who appears to have stage I disease).
What is systematic retroperitoneal lymphadenectomy?

A. Block dissection of common, external and internal iliac and obturator lymph nodes

B. Block dissection of common, external and internal iliac lymph nodes

C. Block dissection of common, external and internal iliac, obturator, lower para-aortic and bifurcation of aorta lymph nodes

D. Block dissection of lymph nodes from the pelvic side walls to the level of the renal veins)

E. Block dissection of the para-aortic lymph nodes

366 NICE recommends that women with suspected stage 1 ovarian cancer should undergo optimal surgical staging.
What is optimal surgical staging?

A. Midline laparotomy to allow thorough assessment of the abdomen and pelvis; a total abdominal hysterectomy, bilateral salpingo-oophorectomy and infracolic omentectomy; biopsies of any peritoneal deposits; random biopsies of the pelvic and abdominal peritoneum; and retroperitoneal lymph node assessment

B. Midline laparotomy to allow thorough assessment of the abdomen and pelvis; a total abdominal hysterectomy, bilateral salpingo-oophorectomy and infracolic omentectomy and retroperitoneal lymph node assessment

C. Midline laparotomy to allow thorough assessment of the abdomen and pelvis; a total abdominal hysterectomy, bilateral salpingo-oophorectomy and infracolic omentectomy; biopsies of any peritoneal deposits; random biopsies of the pelvic and abdominal peritoneum

D. Midline laparotomy to allow thorough assessment of the abdomen and pelvis; a total abdominal hysterectomy, bilateral salpingo-oophorectomy and infracolic omental biopsy; biopsies of any peritoneal deposits; random biopsies of the pelvic and abdominal peritoneum; and retroperitoneal lymph node assessment

E. Midline laparotomy to allow thorough assessment of the abdomen and pelvis; a total abdominal hysterectomy, bilateral salpingo-oophorectomy and infracolic omentectomy; biopsies of any peritoneal deposits; random biopsies of the pelvic and abdominal peritoneum; and systematic retroperitoneal lymphadenectomy

367 A 70-year-old woman underwent optimal surgical staging for suspected early stage ovarian cancer. Her final histology showed stage 1a grade 3 epithelial ovarian cancers.

What is the preferred plan of care after discussion in MDT?

A. Follow-up in 3 months with CT scan and serum Ca125

B. Follow-up in 6 months with CT scan and serum Ca125

C. Offer adjuvant Chemotherapy as 6 cycles of Carboplatin

D. Offer adjuvant Chemotherapy as 6 Cycles of Carboplatin and Bevacizumab

E. Offer adjuvant Chemotherapy as 6 Cycles of Carboplatin and Taxol

368 It is estimated that 75% of women with ovarian cancer currently receive a paclitaxel/platinum combination as first-line therapy.

Although most patients (70–80%) initially respond to first-line chemotherapy, most responders eventually relapse (55–75% within 2 years).

What is the definition of 'Complete response' to chemotherapy ?

A. Malignant disease not detectable for at least 4 weeks

B. Malignant disease not detectable for at least 8 weeks

C. Malignant disease not detectable for at least 12 weeks

D. Malignant disease not detectable for at least 6 months

E. Malignant disease not detectable for at least 12 months

369 A 70-year-old woman has undergone laparotomy for suspected ovarian cancer. At laparotomy, the cancer is found to involve the left ovary and uterus and she has positive peritoneal washings.

As per the FIGO classification for staging of ovarian cancer, what is her staging?

A. Stage IC

B. Stage IIA

C. Stage IIB

D. Stage IIC

E. Stage IIIC

370 A 65-year-old woman complaining of severe itching is diagnosed with Vulval intraepithelial neoplasia (VIN) 3 on biopsy.

What is the first line of management?

A. Laser ablation

B. Local excision

C. Topical cidofir

D. Topical imiquimod

E. Wait and watch

371 A 65-year-old woman presents with a history of vulval discomfort and soreness for 6 months. On examination, there is 2.5 cm raised ulcerated area on the left labia majora which looks highly suspicious of vulval cancer.

What is the first line of investigation?

A. Multiple punch biopsies with adjacent normal skin

B. Sentinel lymph node biopsy

C. Urgent CT scan

D. Urgent MRI

E. Wide local excision biopsy

372 In vulval cancer, the depth of invasion directly correlates with lymph node involvement, thus affecting prognosis and the management plan.

What is the rate of lymph node involvement in women with stage 1a (<1 mm invasion) vulval cancer?

A. <1%

B. 5%

C. 7.5%

D. 10%

E. 25%

373 Vulval cancers are relatively rare cancers with surgery as the mainstay of treatment. In recent years, a lot of emphasis has been given to sentinel node biopsy to decide management.

What is the role of sentinel node biopsy in the management of early vulval cancer?

A. To decide interval of follow-up

B. To decide on the need for lymph node resection

C. To decide on the need for postoperative radiotherapy

D. To evaluate for postoperative chemo radiotherapy

E. To evaluate the need for radical vulvectomy

374 Vulval cancers account for 6% of gynaecological cancers in the United Kingdom. In 2009, a new FIGO staging was introduced with greater emphasis on the inguino-femoral lymph node status to understand prognosis.

What is the FIGO stage for a woman who has a 3 cm vulval cancer involving the anus with metastases in 2 lymph nodes <5 mm?

A. Stage IIIa

B. Stage IIIb

C. Stage IIIc

D. Stage IVa

E. Stage IVb

375 Primary vaginal cancer is rare. There were 281 cases of vaginal cancer in the United Kingdom in 2010. The most common causes of squamous cell vaginal cancer are HPV and irradiation.

What is the most common HPV type found in vaginal cancers?

A. HPV 6

B. HPV 11

C. HPV 16

D. HPV 18

E. HPV 31

376 Recently, the prevalence of HPV-related VIN has increased significantly and consequently the incidence of vulval cancer in young women is rising.

What are the most common HPV serotypes found in vulval cancers?

A. HPV 5 and 8

B. HPV 6 and 11

C. HPV 16 and 18

D. HPV 31 and 33

E. HPV 58 and 59

377 A 45-year-old woman complains of intermenstrual bleeding for the past 6 months. Past history includes 6 normal vaginal deliveries and hypertension and last smear was over 5 years ago. On speculum examination, there is a raised 2 cm friable area on the cervix.

What is the most likely diagnosis?

A. Cervical cancer

B. Cervical ectropion

C. Cervical polyp

D. Cervical warts

E. Chlamydia infection

378 A 40-year-old woman with severe dyskariosis on smear underwent colposcopy and large loop excision of transformation zone (LLETZ). Histology confirmed a moderately differentiated squamous cell carcinoma 4 mm deep and 6 mm wide. Clinical and radiological examination confirmed organ confined disease.

What stage of cervical cancer is this?

A. Stage IA1

B. Stage IA2

C. Stage IB1

D. Stage IB2

E. Stage IIA1

379 A 53-year-old woman is diagnosed with stage IA1 cervical squamous cell carcinoma after histological, clinical and radiological assessment.

What is the most appropriate management plan?

A. Conisation

B. Modified radical hysterectomy with removal of lymph nodes

C. Radical trachelectomy

D. Total abdominal hysterectomy with bilateral salpingo-oophorectomy

E. Total abdominal hysterectomy with conservation of ovaries

380 A 35-year-old woman is diagnosed with stage IB1 cervical squamous cell carcinoma of the cervix on histological and clinical assessment.

What is the most appropriate radiological investigation for this patient?

A. CT scan of abdomen and pelvis

B. CT scan of chest, abdomen and pelvis

C. MRI of abdomen and pelvis

D. PET CT scan

E. Ultrasound of abdomen and pelvis

Urogynaecology and Pelvic Floor Problems

381 An 84-year-old patient who had a previous history of vaginal hysterectomy presents with a stage 3 vault prolapse. The patient has limited mobility and has previously had difficulty with the use of vaginal pessaries.

What is the most appropriate treatment option?

A. Abdominal Sacrocolpopexy

B. Colpocliesis

C. Physiotherapy

D. Sacrospinous fixation

E. Transvaginal repair with mesh

382 A 55-year-old patient presents with a history of urinary symptoms of urgency, increased frequency and nocturia. The patient states that she does not have symptoms of hesitancy and feels as though she empties her bladder completely.

What would be the first line of management?

A. Cystoscopy

B. Neuromodulation

C. Reduce caffeine intake and start anticholinergic medication

D. Ultrasound scan to rule out pelvic pathology

E. Urodynamics

Part 2 MRCOG: Single Best Answer Questions, First Edition.
Andrew Sizer, Chandrika Balachandar, Nibedan Biswas, Richard Foon,
Anthony Griffiths, Sheena Hodgett, Banchhita Sahu and Martyn Underwood.

383 A 39-year-old patient presents with symptoms of leakage of urine upon coughing, sneezing and during exercise. The symptoms started following the birth of her second child 18 months ago.

What would be the first line of management?

A. Biofeedback/Electrical stimulation
B. Bladder retraining
C. Insertion of a midurethral retropubic tape
D. Pharmacotherapy with Duloxetine
E. Supervised Pelvic floor muscle training

384 A patient presents as an emergency with urinary retention. Upon taking a history, you also discover that the patient has been having hematuria for several weeks.

What is an absolute contraindication to inserting a suprapubic catheter?

A. Ascites
B. Bladder tumor
C. Clotting disorders
D. History of extensive bladder reconstruction
E. Unable to fill the bladder to a volume excess of 300 ml

385 A 56-year-old para 4 woman presents with a vault prolapse. The patient is sexually active and urodynamic investigations fail to reveal urodynamic stress incontinence even after reduction of the prolapse.

The patient is keen on having surgery.

Which of the following operations should be offered?

A. Bilateral Sacrospinous fixation
B. Sacrocolpopexy
C. Sacrocolpopexy and insertion of a mid urethral retropubic tape
D. Sacrocolpopexy with a Burch Colposuspension
E. Unilateral Sacrospinous fixation with insertion of a mid-urethral retropubic tape

386 A 39-year-old para 1 patient presents with stress incontinence with no other urinary symptoms.

What would be the first line of management?

A. A trial of pelvic floor muscle training for at least 3 months
B. Electric stimulation in combination with pelvic floor muscle training
C. Pelvic floor electromyography (biofeedback)
D. Pelvic floor muscle training that involves 6 contractions done every 3 days for 6 months
E. Urodynamic studies

387 A patient is undergoing a vaginal hysterectomy for uterine prolapse and at the end of the procedure it is noted that the vault of the vagina descends to 3 cm above the hymenal ring.

What should be considered in order to prevent further descent of the vault in the future?

A. McCall culdoplasty

B. Moschowitz-type operation

C. No further action

D. Sacrospinous fixation

E. Suturing the cardinal and uterosacral ligaments to the vaginal cuff

388 A fit and healthy 52-year-old patient with confirmed detrusor overactivity has tried three different medical treatments (Oxybutynin, Solifenacin, Mirabegron).

The procedure that should be offered to the patient is

A. Botulinum toxin A injections into the bladder

B. Detrusor myomectomy

C. Percutaneous tibial nerve stimulation

D. Sacral nerve modulation

E. Urinary diversion

389 A 38-year-old patient is suffering with stress incontinence. Her BMI is 32 kg/m^2 and the patient is interested in lifestyle management for her incontinence.

What is the most important lifestyle change that you would recommend?

A. Avoidance of caffeinated drinks

B. Exercise

C. Reduction of alcohol intake

D. Reduction of fluid intake

E. Weight loss

390 A 38-year-old patient is suffering with symptoms of an overactive bladder. Her BMI is 25kg/m2 and the patient is interested in lifestyle changes.

What is the most important lifestyle change that you would recommend?

A. Avoidance of caffeinated drinks

B. Exercise

C. Reduction of alcohol intake

D. Reduction of fluid intake

E. Weight loss

391 A patient presents with symptoms of a prolapse. On examination, the pelvic organ quantification score is Aa 0, Ba 0, C −5, D −7, Ap −2 Bp −2 tvl 9, gh 4, pb 3.

The patient wants her prolapse to be treated surgically.

What is the correct diagnosis and surgical treatment?

A. Stage 1 cystocele and no treatment needed

B. Stage 2 cystocele and anterior repair

C. Stage 2 rectocele and posterior repair

D. Stage 2 uterine prolapse/cystocele and vaginal hysterectomy and anterior repair

E. Stage 2 uterine prolapse/rectocele and vaginal hysterectomy and posterior repair

392 A woman presents with symptoms of a prolapse. On examination, the pelvic organ quantification score is Aa −2, Ba −2, C −5, D −7, Ap 0 Bp 0 tvl 9, gh 4, pb 3

The patient wants her prolapse to be treated surgically.

What is the correct diagnosis and surgical treatment?

A. Stage 2 cystocele and anterior repair

B. Stage 1 cystocele and no treatment needed

C. Stage 2 rectocele and posterior repair

D. Stage 2 uterine prolapse/cystocele and vaginal hysterectomy and anterior repair

E. Stage 2 uterine prolapse/rectocele and vaginal hysterectomy and posterior repair

393 A 32-year-old multiparous woman has confirmed urodynamic stress incontinence and admits that she has not completed her family.

What management would you propose for this patient?

A. Advice the patient to compete her family before considering incontinence surgery

B. A periurethral bladder neck injection would be the treatment of choice for long-term relief

C. If the patient has had previous incontinence surgery and the incontinence recurs postpartum then await spontaneous recovery for about 3–4 months

D. If the patient has had previous incontinence surgery a Colposuspension is most likely to be safe and effective

E. If the patient insists on surgery an insertion of a midurethral retropubic tape would be the surgical treatment of choice

394 A 28-year-old woman presents with a history of pelvic pain, urinary urgency, increased frequency and nocturia. The pelvic pain tends to occur during bladder filling and is relieved by voiding and you suspect that the patient has interstitial cystitis.

What other mandatory investigation is required in order to make an accurate diagnosis?

A. Cystoscopy
B. Questionnaires and symptom scales
C. Urinalysis
D. Urinary diary
E. Urodynamics

395 A 64-year-old patient presents with a history of increased urinary frequency, nocturia, urgency and occasional urgency incontinence.

What would be the next line of management?

A. Cystoscopy
B. Trial of anticholinergic medication
C. Urinalysis
D. Urinary diary
E. Urodynamics

396 An 84-year-old patient presents with symptoms of urgency, urgency incontinence and nocturia. The patient is taking several different medications for other medical conditions. A diagnosis of overactive bladder is made.

The general practitioner has already tried Oxybutynin but the patient had side effects (central nervous system) and this was stopped.

Which anticholinergic medication would you now consider?

A. Darifenacin
B. Fesotrodine
C. Solifenacin
D. Tolterodine
E. Trospium chloride

397 A 52-year-old patient presents with a history suggestive of an overactive bladder, but also complains of faecal incontinence.

The patient has tried conservative measures and various anticholinergics with no significant benefit.

Urodynamic testing confirms detrusor overactivity and some voiding dysfunction.

What is the best surgical option for this patient?

A. Augmentation cystoplasty

B. Botulinum toxin injections to the bladder and teaching the patient intermittent self-catheterisation

C. Intravesical therapy (Oxybutynin)

D. Posterior tibial nerve stimulation

E. Sacral neuromodulation

398 You have just completed a vaginal hysterectomy for a procedentia. However, upon catheterisation, no urine is present in the catheter bag.

A cystoscopy is performed and no bladder trauma is identified. In order to assess ureteric function you give indigo carmine and after 5 minutes you observe a blue stream from the right ureteric orifice but none from the left.

What would be the next line of management?

A. Contact the urologist with a view to stenting the ureter

B. Cut the sutures that you used for vault support and see if there is any change in your cystoscopy findings

C. Give an intravenous a bolus dose of a diuretic and wait another 5–10 minutes

D. Insert a catheter into the bladder and perform postoperative imaging

E. Perform an intra operative ultrasound

399 A 48-year-old morbidly obese woman has a sister who recently had surgical treatment for prolapse.

She is therefore interested in finding more about the impact of obesity on the development of prolapse.

The occurrence of which type of prolapse shows the most significant increase in association with morbid obesity?

A. Cystocele

B. Enterocele

C. Rectocele

D. Urethral prolapse

E. Uterine prolapse

400 A woman is contemplating having either a Sacrospinouscolpopexy (no mesh) or a Sacrocolpopexy (with mesh).

The patient is keen on having a Sacrocolpopexy but is concerned about novo prolapse.

What is the incidence of de novo prolapse (cystocele), after Sacrocolpopexy and Sacrospinouscolpopexy?

	Sacrocolpopexy	Sacrospinouscolpopexy
A.	2%	4%
B.	8%	8%
C.	14%	12%
D.	24%	12%
E.	31%	14%

Explanations

Module 3

IT, Governance and Research

1 If involved in a serious incident requiring investigation (SIRI), initial steps would involve completing an incident form, ensuring completion of notes accurately and participating in team debrief.

If a trainee is involved in an SIRI, what action should be taken as soon as possible?

A. Discuss with the medical defence organisation

B. Engage fully with the investigation

C. Meet with the educational supervisor to discuss the case

D. Write a formal statement

E. Write a reflection of the vent

TOG Article

Macdonald M, Gosakan R, Cooper AE, Fothergill DJ. Dealing with a serious incident requiring investigation in obstetrics and gynaecology: a training perspective. The Obstetrician & Gynaecologist 2014;16:109–114.

An early reporting system ensures that trainees get the right support and they are advised to meet with their educational supervisor as soon as possible to discuss the case.

2 In surrogacy arrangement, the commissioning couple need to obtain parental orders. Within what time frame after delivery must these be made?

A. 6 months

B. 12 months

C. 18 months

D. 24 months

E. 36 months

Part 2 MRCOG: Single Best Answer Questions, First Edition.
Andrew Sizer, Chandrika Balachandar, Nibedan Biswas, Richard Foon,
Anthony Griffiths, Sheena Hodgett, Banchhita Sahu and Martyn Underwood.
© 2016 John Wiley & Sons, Ltd. Published 2016 by John Wiley & Sons, Ltd.

TOG Article

Burrell C, O'Connor H. Surrogate pregnancy: ethical and medico-legal issues in modern obstetrics. The Obstetrician & Gynaecologist 2013;15:113–119.

Under the HFE Act 20086 section 54, parental orders are granted if:

- The commissioning couple are married, in a civil partnership or cohabitees and both are >18 years old.
- The conception must be from placing the embryo, sperm or egg into the surrogate mother or by donor insemination. The egg or sperm must be from one member of the commissioning couple, thus providing a genetic link.
- The application must be made within 6 months after delivery.
- The child must be living with the commissioning couple, one or both of whom must be domiciled in the United Kingdom.
- The surrogate (and the legal father if not the commissioning father) must give consent for the parental order transfer within 6 weeks after delivery.
- No payment should be made to the surrogate (other than reasonable expenses). Expenses are decided by the court.

3 When managing a patient with surrogate pregnancy, who decides about the treatment required for any clinical situation that may affect the pregnancy?
A. The binding agreement
B. The commissioning father
C. The commissioning mother
D. The surrogate mother
E. The unborn child

TOG Article

Burrell C, O'Connor H. Surrogate pregnancy: ethical and medico-legal issues in modern obstetrics. The Obstetrician & Gynaecologist 2013;15:113–119.

A duty of care is owed to the surrogate mother. The unborn fetus has no legal rights, so the surrogate must make all decisions, even if it is not in the best interests of the fetus (including lawful termination). In the event of conflict, the surrogate should be supported to make the final decision without coercion.

4 A primigravida at 24 weeks gestation has come to the antenatal clinic with a fear of childbirth and is asking for elective caesarean section as a mode of delivery.

What would be the recommended management?

A. Adequate exploration of the fears with counselling by trained personnel

B. Discharging the patient to midwife care with advise for vaginal delivery

C. Enlisting the patient for elective caesarean section

D. Referral to another obstetrician for second opinion

E. Referral to the supervisor of midwife

TOG Article

Nama V, Wilcock F. Caesarean section on maternal request: is justification necessary? The Obstetrician & Gynaecologist 2011;13:263–269.

Rather than counselling women requesting caesarean section about the risks, a better approach would be to explore the reasons for the request. Women who present with fear of childbirth have serious concerns about birth and related issues. Adequate exploration of the fears, together with counselling, has been shown to alleviate them. The factors that can predispose these women to develop PTSD should be identified and addressed. Frequent, regular psychotherapy by trained personnel to address tokophobia for women who request caesarean section is likely to result in almost half of these women ultimately choosing a vaginal delivery.

5 Women requesting caesarean section on maternal request might have posttraumatic stress disorder (PTSD) after previous childbirth. What is the incidence of PTSD after childbirth?

A. 0–1%

B. 6–7%

C. 12–13%

D. 24–25%

E. 36–37%

TOG Article

Nama V, Wilcock F. Caesarean section on maternal request: is justification necessary? The Obstetrician & Gynaecologist 2011;13:263–269.

Women who request caesarean section or who have a deep fear of childbirth are known to have lower socialisation scores and higher levels of anxiety and are more likely to have depressive symptomatology. These are the risk factors for pre-traumatic stress disorder and PTSD. The general incidence of PTSD after childbirth is 6–7%; the most important predictors are emergency caesarean section and instrumental vaginal delivery, which can persist for up to 2 years.

6 Among those receiving gynaecological treatment, what is the reported incidence of domestic violence in the United Kingdom?

A. 11%
B. 21%
C. 31%
D. 41%
E. 51%

TOG Article

Gottlieb AS. Domestic violence: a clinical guide for women's health care providers. The Obstetrician & Gynaecologist 2012;14:197–202.

Domestic violence is a threatening behaviour, violence or abuse (psychological, physical, sexual, financial, emotional) between adults who are or have been intimate partners. The majority of victims are women; population studies estimate that at least one in four women worldwide will be abused by a partner during her lifetime. Clinical research in the United Kingdom demonstrates that 13–24% of women receiving antenatal or postnatal care and 21% of women receiving gynaecological services report a history of domestic violence.

7 When obtaining consent for a procedure, a doctor should take reasonable care in communicating with the patients, as their inability to recall from such discussion is often evident.

What percentage of the information that is discussed during the process of obtaining consent before surgery is retained at 6 months?

A. 10%
B. 20%
C. 30%
D. 40%
E. 50%

TOG Article

Leigh B. Making decisions together, or wake me up when it is over? The Obstetrician & Gynaecologist 2009;11:117–121.

The authors of the different studies asked them at various intervals what they could remember and the results suggested that, by and large, recall was very poor. In one series the patients could remember at 6 months only 10% of what they had been told before they underwent surgery.

8 One of the main challenges faced by clinical trials is a lower than expected rate of recruitment.

What is the key to successful recruitment?

A. Collaboration and collective effort in multicentric trials

B. Do nothing, as clinical trials are not important

C. Provide incentives for participation in medical studies

D. Wait for colleagues to publish clinical trials

E. Withhold care to patients if they do not agree to participate in clinical trials

TOG Article

Thangaratinam S, Khan KS. Participation in research as a means of improving quality of care: the role of a principal investigator in multi-centre clinical trials. The Obstetrician & Gynaecologist 2015;17:55–61.

One of the main challenges faced by clinical studies, both nationally and internationally, is the lower than expected rates of recruitment. One of the keys to successful recruitment is collaboration and collective effort. Furthermore, multicentre studies increase the applicability of the findings across a wide spectrum of settings, and circumvent the criticism that research conclusions are restricted only to those women who were recruited from a single centre.

9 Improved outcomes are often observed in women participating in a clinical trial.

What is the reason behind this improved outcome, irrespective of study findings?

A. Positive change in the behaviour of clinicians and participants along with improved delivery of care

B. There is no difference in the outcome of care

C. Treatment is provided in a new hospital with latest technology

D. Treatment is provided in a tertiary hospital

E. Treatment is usually based on postal delivery of medication

TOG Article

Thangaratinam S, Khan KS. Participation in research as a means of improving quality of care: the role of a principal investigator in multi-centre clinical trials. The Obstetrician & Gynaecologist 2015;17:55–61.

The improved outcomes observed in the women involved in a clinical trial, irrespective of the study findings, may be due to the following reasons: positive change in the behaviour of the clinician or the participant due to the perception of being observed; improved delivery of care such as prompt action on the laboratory results or better nursing care by virtue of being in a trial; compliance with the research protocol within set guidelines leading to improved outcomes;

exposure to a new intervention that may be potentially beneficial; and involvement of motivated clinicians who may also have better clinical expertise, thereby improving the care of women. Research active settings are thus likely to have better outcomes and the percentage of women accrued into studies can be used as a target for service evaluation.

10 On completing a consent form with a patient for a diagnostic laparoscopy, you mention that the chances of suffering a bowel injury is 'uncommon'.

How would you define 'uncommon' in this context in numerical terms?

A. 1/1–1/10
B. 1/10–1/100
C. 1/100–1/1000
D. 1/1000–1/10,000
E. <1/10,000

CGA 6 Obtaining Valid Consent

Table 1. Presenting information on risk

Term	Equivalent numerical ratio	Colloquial equivalent
Very common	1/1 to 1/10	A person in family
Common	1/10 to 1/100	A person in street
Uncommon	1/100 to 1/1000	A person in village
Rare	1/1000 to 1/10 000	A person in small town
Very rare	Less than 1/10 000	A person in large town

Core Surgical Skills

11 A medical student asks you how to measure blood pressure.
What maximum pressure should you inflate the cuff to measure systolic blood pressure in pregnancy?

A. Always initially inflate to 200 mmHg then deflate
B. Patient's palpated diastolic blood pressure
C. Patient's palpated systolic blood pressure
D. Patients palpated systolic blood pressure + 20–30 mmHg
E. Patients palpated systolic blood pressure + 5 mmHg

NICE CG 62 Antenatal Care

Blood pressure should be measured as outlined below:-

- Remove tight clothing, ensure arm is relaxed and supported at heart level
- Use cuff of appropriate size
- Inflate cuff to 20–30 mmHg above palpated systolic blood pressure
- Lower column slowly, by 2 mmHg per second or per beat, read blood pressure to the nearest 2 mmHg
- Measure diastolic blood pressure as disappearance of sounds (phase V).

12 A healthy 39-year-old woman with no significant past medical history attends a preoperative assessment clinic.
She is due to undergo a total abdominal hysterectomy for heavy menstrual bleeding following a local anaesthetic endometrial ablation that was unsuccessful.
She is fit and well.
What preoperative investigation is required?

A. Chest X-ray
B. Coagulation screen
C. Electrocardiogram
D. Full blood count
E. Renal function tests

Part 2 MRCOG: Single Best Answer Questions, First Edition.
Andrew Sizer, Chandrika Balachandar, Nibedan Biswas, Richard Foon, Anthony Griffiths, Sheena Hodgett, Banchhita Sahu and Martyn Underwood.
© 2016 John Wiley & Sons, Ltd. Published 2016 by John Wiley & Sons, Ltd.

NICE CG3 Preoperative Tests
ASA Grade 1: adults ≥ 16 years

Test	Age (years)			
	≥ 16 to < 40	≥ 40 to < 60	≥ 60 to < 80	≥ 80
Chest X-ray	No	No	Consider	Consider
ECG	No	Consider	Yes	Yes
Full blood count	Yes	Yes	Yes	Yes
Haemostasis	No	No	No	No
Renal function	Consider	Consider	Yes	Yes
Random glucose	Consider	Consider	Consider	Consider
Urine analysis[a]	Consider	Consider	Consider	Consider

13 On deciding where to place your secondary lateral ports at laparoscopy, care should be taken to avoid the inferior epigastric vessels.

Where can these be found?

A. ~2cm from the midline

B. Lateral to the lateral umbilical ligaments

C. Lateral to the medial umbilical ligaments

D. Medial to the lateral umbilical ligaments

E. Medial to the medial umbilical ligaments

GTG 49 Preventing Entry-Related Gynaecological Laparoscopic Injuries

The deep epigastric arteries and the venae comitantes running beside them can be visualised just lateral to the lateral umbilical ligaments (the obliterated hypogastric arteries) in all but the most obese patient.

14 Your hospital has recently had an increase in postoperative infections. As a result, you are formulating a new guideline that includes information on skin preparation and hair removal prior to surgery. What is the most appropriate method of hair removal prior to surgery?

A. **Electric clippers**
B. Electrolysis
C. Laser
D. Shaving
E. Waxing

NICE CG 74 Surgical Site Infection: Prevention and Treatment of Surgical Site Infection

If hair has to be removed, use electric clippers with a single-use head on the day of surgery. Do not use razors for hair removal, because they increase the risk of surgical-site infection.

15 Following delivery, a woman is found to have a third degree tear and a trainee wishes to do the repair under supervision.

Which two suture materials have equivalent efficacy when repairing the external anal sphincter?

A. Polydiaxanone (PDS) and chromic catgut
B. Polydiaxanone (PDS) and nylon (Prolene)
C. **Polydiaxanone (PDS) and Polyglactin (Vicryl)**
D. Polyglactin (Vicryl and chromic catgut
E. Polyglactin (Vicryl) and nylon (Prolene)

GTG 29 The Management of Third and Fourth Degree Perineal Tears

Option c is the only option supported by Grade A evidence

16 A 45-year-old woman is undergoing an abdominal hysterectomy for a history of heavy menstrual bleeding that has not responded to medical treatment. The patient has a past history of pelvic pain and the operation notes from a previous laparoscopy comments that the patient had 'pelvic adhesions'

What is the most appropriate action in terms of protecting the ureter?

A. **Identify the ureter tracing it from the pelvic brim and mobilise the ureter by incising the peritoneum and sweeping the tissues laterally**
B. Mobilise the entire ureter with the aid of electrosurgery to reduce the blood loss
C. Perform a preoperative MRI
D. Perform a preoperative MRI and Intravenous urogram to assess the ureters
E. Perform preoperative ureteric stenting

TOG Article

Minas V, Gul N, Aust T, Doyle M, Rowlands D. Urinary tract injuries in laparoscopic gynaecological surgery; prevention, recognition and management. The Obstetrician & Gynaecologist 2014;16:19–28.

Performing an MRI with or without an intravenous urogram preoperatively is not recommended. Preoperative stenting has shown to have no significant benefit and is only used in selective cases. One should avoid using electrosurgery close to the ureter as it can cause thermal injuries.

17 A 45-year-old asthmatic patient attends the gynaecology clinic with heavy menstrual bleeding and an ultrasound scan suggests the presence of an endometrial polyp.

The patient is booked for an outpatient hysteroscopy.

What analgesia should be prescribed at least 1 hour before the procedure?

A. Buprenorphine

B. Diclofenac

C. Ibuprofen

D. Paracetamol

E. Tramadol

GTG 59 Best Practice in Outpatient Hysteroscopy

Routine use of opiate analgesia before outpatient hysteroscopy should be avoided as it may cause adverse effects.

Women without contraindications should be advised to consider taking standard doses of non-steroidal anti-inflammatory agents (NSAIDs) around 1 hour before their scheduled outpatient hysteroscopy appointment with the aim of reducing pain in the immediate postoperative period.

Paracetamol and NSAIDS can both be used but as the patient is asthmatic, probably it would be better to avoid NSAIDS.

18 What is the preferred distension medium for outpatient diagnostic hysteroscopy?

A. Carbon dioxide

B. Dextran

C. Glycine

D. Icodextrin

E. Normal saline

GTG 59 Best Practice in Outpatient Hysteroscopy

Uterine distension with normal saline allows improved image quality and allows outpatient diagnostic hysteroscopy to be completed more quickly as compared with uterine distension with carbon dioxide.

19 At what pressure should the pneumoperitoneum be maintained during the insertion of secondary ports for a laparoscopic procedure?

A. 5–10 mmHg

B. 12–15 mmHg

C. 20–25 mmHg

D. 30–35 mmHg

E. >35 mmHg

GTG 49 Preventing Entry-Related Gynaecological Laparoscopic Injuries

Secondary ports must be inserted under direct vision perpendicular to the skin, while maintaining the pneumoperitoneum at 20–25 mmHg.

20 What is the background rate of venous thromboembolism in healthy non-pregnant non-contraceptive using women?

A. 0.5/10,000/year

B. 2/10,000/year

C. 5/10,000/year

D. 10/10,000/year

E. 20/10,000/year

FSRH Statement Venous Thromboembolism (VTE) and Hormonal Contraception

Table 2: Risk of venous thromboembolism (VTE) associated with non-use, combined hormonal contraception (CHC) use over the course of 1 year (adapted from http://www.ema.europa.eu/ema/index.jsp?curl=pages/news_and_events/news/2013/11/news_detail_001969.jsp&mid=WC0b01ac058004d5c1)

	Risk of VTE per 10,000 healthy women over one year
Non contraceptive users and not pregnant	2
CHC containing ethinylestradiol plus levonorgestrel, norgestimate or norethisterone	5-7
CHC containing etonogestrel (ring) or norelgestromin (patch)	6-12
CHC containing ethinylestradiol plus gestodene, desogestrel or drospirenone	9-12

Module 6

Postoperative Care

21 What proportion of patients having a surgical procedure will develop a surgical site infection?
   A. 5%
   B. 10%
   C. 15%
   D. 20%
   E. 25%

NICE CG74 Surgical Site Infection

Surgical site infections have been shown to compose up to 20% of all of health care-associated infections. At least 5% of patients undergoing a surgical procedure develop a surgical site infection.

22 What is the most common source of microorganisms causing surgical site infection?
   A. Anaesthetist
   B. Contaminated surgical equipment
   C. Patient
   D. Postoperative nursing staff
   E. Surgeon

NICE CG74 Surgical Site Infection

Most surgical site infections are caused by contamination of an incision by microorganisms from the patient's own body during surgery. Infection caused by microorganisms from an outside source following surgery is less common.

Part 2 MRCOG: Single Best Answer Questions, First Edition.
Andrew Sizer, Chandrika Balachandar, Nibedan Biswas, Richard Foon, Anthony Griffiths, Sheena Hodgett, Banchhita Sahu and Martyn Underwood.
© 2016 John Wiley & Sons, Ltd. Published 2016 by John Wiley & Sons, Ltd.

23 A 54-year-old patient has had an insertion of a mid urethral retropubic tape and following the procedure there was a significant fall in the haemoglobin levels from 12.3 g/dl to 7.8 g/dl. Imaging investigations show the presence of retropubic hematoma. A decision is made to evacuate the hematoma. The most appropriate incision would be:

A. Cherney incision

B. Kustner incision

C. Maylard incision

D. Midline (median) incision

E. Pfannenstiel incision

TOG Article

Raghavan R, Arya P, Arya P, China S. Abdominal incisions and sutures in obstetrics and Gynaecology. The Obstetrician & Gynaecologist 2014;16:13–18

The Cherney incision allows access to the retropubic area (space of Retzius) and also the pelvic sidewall in order to evacuate and identify the source of the bleeding.

24 A postoperative patient who had a hysterectomy received morphine in recovery and then again in the gynaecology ward. Her respiratory rate is suppressed; she is drowsy and has pinpoint pupils.

What medication would you give to reverse this potential morphine overdose?

A. Atropine

B. Buprenorphine

C. Flumazenil

D. Naloxone

E. Pethidine

BNF Online Section 15.1.7

NALOXONE HYDROCHLORIDE

Indications

Overdosage with opioids; reversal of postoperative respiratory depression and reversal of neonatal respiratory and CNS depression resulting from opioid administration to mother during labur.

25 A patient who is frail, old and overweight has undergone a midline laparotomy and pelvic clearance for an endometrial cancer.

On postoperative day 4, the nursing staff notice that she has a pressure ulcer with full thickness skin loss, but the bone, tendon and muscle are not exposed.

What type of pressure ulcer grade is this?

A. Grade 1

B. Grade 2

C. Grade 3

D. Grade 4

E. Grade 5

http://nhs.stopthepressure.co.uk/docs/ PU-Grading-Chart.pdf

EPUAP – Category/Grade 3

Full thickness skin loss. Subcutaneous fat may be visible but bone, tendon and muscle are not exposed.

May include undermining and tunnelling.

The depth varies by anatomical location (bridge of the nose, ear, occiput and malleolus do not have (adipose) subcutaneous tissue and grade 3 ulcers can be shallow.

In contrast, area of significant adiposity can develop extremely deep grade 3 pressure ulcers.

Bone/tendon is not visible or is directly palpable.

26 A woman had an emergency caesarean section for a pathological CTG and pyrexia in labour. She was discharged on postoperative day 4 but re-admitted on day 6 with pyrexia, tachypnoea, tachycardia and hypotension. Haemoglobin is 105 g/l.

Septic shock is the main differential diagnosis.

Following the Sepsis 6 bundle, along with antibiotics and blood cultures, which other important blood test needs to be taken?

A. C-Reactive protein

B. Fibrinogen

C. Lactate

D. Urea and electrolytes

E. White Cell Count

http://survivesepsis.org/the-sepsis-six/

The Sepsis Six are:

1. Administer high flow oxygen
2. Take blood cultures
3. Give broad spectrum antibiotics
4. Give intravenous fluid challenges
5. Measure serum lactate and haemoglobin
6. Measure accurate hourly urine output.

27 A patient undergoes a challenging hysterectomy. A drain is left in the pelvis. You are called to review the patient eight hours later as the nurses have noted a high serous drain output and poor urinary output.

What finding would identify if the drain fluid is urine (suggestive of a bladder/ureteric injury) or normal peritoneal fluid?

A. Peritoneal creatinine > urine nitrogen

B. Peritoneal urea > urine urea

C. Serum creatinine > peritoneal creatinine

D. Serum nitrogen > drain fluid nitrogen levels

E. Urine nitrogen > peritoneal nitrogen

Journal Article

Manahan KJ, Fanning J. Peritoneal fluid urea nitrogen and creatinine reference values. Obstet Gynecol. 1999;93,5:780–782.

Normal reference values of urea nitrogen and creatinine in peritoneal fluid are equivalent to serum values and are significantly less than urine levels.

Urea nitrogen and creatinine values are found to be significantly higher in urine (47–157 times greater) compared to serum and normal peritoneal fluid.

If you take fluid from an abdominal or pelvic drain that you suspect may be urine, measure the urea nitrogen and creatinine values, and if they are all significantly increased this suggests that the fluid is urine and not peritoneal and that it is coming from a bladder or ureteric injury.

28 A patient has a ventouse delivery. Two days later she reports general malaise, fever and feeling unwell.

With sepsis, which is the first clinical sign to deteriorate, which can be detected through the use of early warning scores?

A. Altered consciousness

B. Hypotension

C. Hypoxia

D. Tachycardia

E. Tachypnoea

Web Article

Assenzio B, Martin-Conte EL. Cellular Mechanisms of MOF During Severe Sepsis and Septic Shock, Severe Sepsis and Septic Shock - Understanding a Serious Killer, Dr Ricardo Fernandez (Ed.), 2012;

ISBN: 978-953-307-950-9, InTech, DOI: 10.5772/27398. Available from: http://www.intechopen.com/books/severe-sepsis-and-septic-shock-understanding-a-serious-killer/cellular-mechanisms-of-mof-during-septic-shock

Tachypnoea is often the first detectable clinical sign of developing sepsis for several reasons. Rapid breathing can be caused by fever, lactic acidosis, pulmonary edema and because the lungs are the most common site of infection. In addition, the lung is often the first organ to undergo dysfunction during sepsis due to its early involvement in the inflammatory process. This can lead to acute lung injury (ALI) or acute respiratory distress syndrome (ARDS).

29 Oral fluids and food are often delayed following major gynaecological surgery.

Which gastrointestinal complication is improved by early postoperative feeding?

A. Abdominal distension

B. Incidence of diarrhoea

C. Need for nasogastric tube placement

D. Recovery of bowel function

E. Rectal bleeding

Cochrane Review

Charoenkwan K, Matovinovic E. Early versus delayed oral fluids and food for reducing complications after major abdominal gynecologic surgery. Cochrane Database of Systematic Reviews 2014, Issue 12.

There was no evidence of a difference between the study groups in abdominal distension or a need for postoperative nasogastric tube placement. Early feeding was associated with shorter time to the presence of bowel sound and faster onset of flatus. Early postoperative feeding after major abdominal gynaecologic surgery appeared to be safe without increased gastrointestinal morbidities or other postoperative complications. The benefits of this approach include faster recovery of bowel function, lower rates of infectious complications, shorter hospital stay and higher satisfaction.

30 Following a difficult hysterectomy, a 65-year old woman has returned to the gynaecology ward. She had large amounts of morphine in the recovery area for pain relief and is also connected to a patient-controlled analgesia device.

The nurses note that she is drowsy and her respiratory rate is low.

The anesthetist decides to perform arterial blood gas sampling. What disturbance of acid–base balance is this most likely to show?

A. Metabolic acidosis

B. Metabolic alkalosis

C. No disturbance

D. Respiratory acidosis

E. Respiratory alkalosis

Journal Article

Epstein SK, Singh N. Respiratory acidosis. Respir Care. 2001; 46:366–383.

Respiratory acidosis, or primary hypercapnia, is the acid–base disorder that results from an increase in arterial partial pressure of carbon dioxide. Acute respiratory acidosis occurs with acute (Type II) respiratory failure, which can result from any sudden respiratory parenchymal (e.g., pulmonary edema), airways (e.g., chronic obstructive pulmonary disease or asthma), pleural, chest wall, neuromuscular (e.g., spinal cord injury) or central nervous system event (e.g., drug overdose).

Module 7

Surgical Procedures

31 Which type of ureteric injury is most commonly reported at laparoscopy?

A. Crush
B. Laceration
C. Ligation
D. Thermal
E. Transection

TOG Article

Minas V, Gul N, Aust T, Doyle M, Rowlands D. Urinary tract injuries in laparoscopic gynaecological surgery; prevention, recognition and management. The Obstetrician & Gynaecologist 2014;16:19–28.

There are seven types of ureteric injury with transection being the most commonly reported at laparoscopy.

32 During laparoscopic pelvic surgery, which visceral structure is most likely to be damaged?

A. Aorta
B. Bladder
C. Ileum
D. Rectum
E. Ureter

TOG Article

Minas V, Gul N, Aust T, Doyle M, Rowlands D. Urinary tract injuries in laparoscopic gynaecological surgery; prevention, recognition and management. The Obstetrician & Gynaecologist, 2014;16:19–28.

Part 2 MRCOG: Single Best Answer Questions, First Edition.
Andrew Sizer, Chandrika Balachandar, Nibedan Biswas, Richard Foon,
Anthony Griffiths, Sheena Hodgett, Banchhita Sahu and Martyn Underwood.
© 2016 John Wiley & Sons, Ltd. Published 2016 by John Wiley & Sons, Ltd.

Injury rates range from 0.02% to 8.3% placing bladder injury at the top of the list of visceral damage complications related to laparoscopic pelvic surgery.

33 Theoretically, what kind of injury related to laparoscopic entry should be reduced by the Hasson (open) technique, compared to a Veress needle entry?

A. Bladder injury

B. Bowel injury

C. Major vessel injury

D. Splenic injury

E. Ureteric injury

GTG 49 Preventing Entry-Related Gynaecological Laparoscopic Injuries

In a meta-analysis of over 350,000 closed laparoscopic procedures, the risk of bowel damage was 0.4/1000 and of major vessel injuries was 0.2/1000. It is anticipated that the open (Hasson) technique would be less likely to cause major vessel injury than the closed method.

34 An 18-year-old nulliparous girl presents as a gynaecological emergency with severe left-sided pelvic pain, tachycardia and vomiting. A pregnancy test is negative. An ultrasound scan is performed in the emergency department, which appears to demonstrate a left adnexal cyst.

In theatre, a laparoscopy is performed which shows an ovarian torsion that has twisted three times on its pedicle. The left tube and ovary appear purple and congested.

What is the most appropriate surgical management?

A. Convert to laparotomy and perform a left salpingo-oophorectomy

B. Laparoscopic left salpingo-oophorectomy

C. Untwist the tube and ovary and perform a laparoscopic ovarian cystectomy

D. Untwist the tube and ovary and perform a oophoropexy

E. Untwist the tube and ovary, drain the ovarian cyst and leave the tube and ovary in situ

TOG Article

Damigos E, Johns J, Ross J. An update on the diagnosis and management of ovarian torsion. The Obstetrician & Gynaecologist 2012;14:229–236.

'..there are good outcome data to support conservative management with laparoscopic de-torsion in the majority of cases with little short or long-term associated morbidity, even if the ovary appears dark purple or black ... '

' ... Whether or not to perform oophoropexy when de-torsion of normal adnexae is performed is less clear ... '

'..In cases where torsion has occurred in the presence of a true ovarian cyst, cystectomy at the time of de-torsion is often risky due to the friable nature of the tissues, but early elective cystectomy has been described after an interval of 2–3 weeks to allow time for the edema and congestion to resolve. In all cases of adnexal torsion, the laparoscopic approach would be the preferred route in order to reduce admission time, postoperative pain and long-term risk of adhesion formation ... '

35 A patient undergoes a laparoscopic cystectomy for a dermoid cyst and some spillage of the contents occurs into the peritoneal cavity. What will be the incidence of chemical peritonitis?

A. **5%**
B. 15%
C. 25%
D. 35%
E. 45%

TOG Article

Stavroulis A, Memtsa M, Yoong W. Methods for specimen removal from the peritoneal cavity after laparoscopic excision. The Obstetrician and Gynaecologist 2013;15:26–30.

Chemical peritonitis is a complication of dermoid cyst spillage with an incidence rate of 0.2–8.0%. The spillage rates of dermoid cysts are reported to be between 15 and 100 % when removed via laparoscopy and 4–13% when removed via laparotomy. Currently, closure of fascia of port sites greater than 5 mm is recommended

36 When comparing robotic-assisted surgery to conventional laparoscopic surgery for gynaecological procedures, what would be the major drawback?

A. Intraoperative complication rate
B. Length of hospital stay
C. **Operative time**
D. Postoperative complication rate
E. Safety and effectiveness in gynaecological cancer

Cochrane Review

Liu H, Lawrie TA, Lu D, Song H, Wang L, Shi G. Robot-assisted surgery in gynaecology. Cochrane Database of Systematic Reviews 2014, Issue 12. Art. No.: CD011422. DOI: 10.1002/14651858.CD011422.

There is uncertainty as to whether robotic-assisted surgery or Conventional Laparoscopic Surgery has lower intraoperative and postoperative complication rates because of the imprecision of the effect and inconsistency among studies. Moderate-quality evidence suggests that these procedures take longer with robotic-assisted surgery but may be associated with a shorter hospital stay following hysterectomy. There is limited evidence on the effectiveness and safety of robotic-assisted surgery compared with conventional laparoscopic surgery performed for gynaecological cancer.

37 A 19-year-old is undergoing a laparoscopy for pelvic pain

What is the estimated risk of death due to a patient undergoing a laparoscopy?

A. 1 in 100
B. 1 in 1000
C. 1 in 10,000
D. 1 in 100,000
E. 1 in 1,000,000

GTG 41 The Initial Management of Chronic Pelvic Pain

Diagnostic laparoscopy is the only test capable of reliably diagnosing peritoneal endometriosis and adhesions. Gynaecologists have therefore seen it as an essential tool in the assessment of women with chronic pelvic pain. However, it carries significant risks: an estimated risk of death of approximately 1 in 10,000, and a risk of injury to bowel, bladder or blood vessel of approximately 2.4 in 1000, of whom two-thirds will require laparotomy.

38 A 22-year-old is undergoing a laparoscopy for suspected endometriosis.

What is the estimated risk of bowel, bladder or blood vessel injury?

A. 1.2:10,000
B. 2.4:10,000
C. 1.2:1000
D. 2.4:1000
E. 4.8:1000

GTG 41 GTG The Initial Management of Chronic Pelvic Pain

Diagnostic laparoscopy is the only test capable of reliably diagnosing peritoneal endometriosis and adhesions. Gynaecologists have therefore seen it as an essential tool in the assessment of women with chronic pelvic pain. However, it carries significant risks: an estimated risk of death of approximately 1 in 10,000, and a risk of injury to bowel, bladder or blood vessel of approximately 2.4 in 1000, of whom two-thirds will require laparotomy.

39 Consent is being obtained from a 24-year-old for a diagnostic laparoscopy and it is correctly documented that there is a risk of laparotomy if any injury to bowel, bladder or blood vessels were to occur during the procedure.

The patient wishes to know what proportion of cases would be converted to a laparotomy should an injury occur?

A. 17%
B. 31%
C. 48%
D. 67%
E. 92%

GTG 41 GTG The Initial Management of Chronic Pelvic Pain

Diagnostic laparoscopy is the only test capable of reliably diagnosing peritoneal endometriosis and adhesions. Gynaecologists have therefore seen it as an essential tool in the assessment of women with chronic pelvic pain. However, it carries significant risks: an estimated risk of death of approximately 1 in 10,000, and a risk of injury to bowel, bladder or blood vessel of approximately 2.4 in 1000, of which two-thirds will require laparotomy.

40 A healthy 54-year-old lady is due to attend the outpatient postmenopausal bleeding hysteroscopy clinic.

Which medication should she be advised to consider taking prior to her attendance at the clinic?

A. Benzodiazepines
B. non-steroidal anti-inflammatory agents (NSAIDs)
C. Opioids
D. Paracetamol
E. Prostaglandins

GTG 59 Best Practice in Outpatient Hysteroscopy

Routine use of opiate analgesia before outpatient hysteroscopy should be avoided as it may cause adverse effects.

Women without contraindications should be advised to consider taking standard doses of non-steroidal anti-inflammatory agents (NSAIDs) around 1 hour before their scheduled outpatient hysteroscopy appointment with the aim of reducing pain in the immediate postoperative period.

41 A 62-year-old is due to undergo a hysteroscopy due to a thickened endometrium detected as part of her investigations for postmenopausal bleeding.
Which medication should be used to 'prime' the cervix prior to the hysteroscopy?
A. Mifepristone
B. Misoprostol
C. No medication required
D. Non-steroidal anti-inflammatory
E. Vaginal oestrogen

GTG 59 Best Practice in Outpatient Hysteroscopy

Routine cervical preparation before outpatient hysteroscopy should not be used in the absence of any evidence of benefit in terms of reduction of pain, rates of failure or uterine trauma.

42 A 43-year-old lady with a history of heavy menstrual bleeding and a scan suggesting a polyp is due to undergo an outpatient hysteroscopy.
Which distension medium is routinely recommended due to its improved quality of image and speed of the procedure?
A. Carbon dioxide
B. Gelofusin
C. Normal saline 0.9%
D. Purosol
E. 5% Glucose

GTG 59 Best Practice in Outpatient Hysteroscopy

For routine outpatient hysteroscopy, the choice of distension medium between carbon dioxide and normal saline should be left to the discretion of the operator as neither is superior in reducing pain, although uterine distension with normal saline appears to reduce the incidence of vasovagal episodes.

Uterine distension with normal saline allows improved image quality and allows outpatient diagnostic hysteroscopy to be completed more quickly compared with uterine distention with carbon dioxide.

Operative outpatient hysteroscopy, using bipolar electro surgery, requires the use of normal saline to act as both the distension and conducting medium.

43 A 32 year old is due to undergo a laparoscopic operation for investigation and management of an ovarian cyst detected on scan.

What is the expected serious complication rate following a laparoscopy?

A. 1:500
B. 1:1000
C. 1:2500
D. 1:5000
E. 1:10,000

GTG 49 Preventing Entry-Related Gynaecological Laparoscopic Injuries

Approximately, 250,000 women undergo laparoscopic surgery in the United Kingdom each year. The majority are without problems but serious complications occur in about 1 in 1000 cases. Laparoscopic injuries frequently occur during the blind insertion of needles, trocars and cannula through the abdominal wall and, hence, the period of greatest risk is from the start of the procedure until visualisation within the peritoneal cavity has been established.

44 With respect to instrumentation of the uterus, which operation has the highest risk of perforation?

A. Division of intrauterine adhesions
B. Outpatient hysteroscopy
C. Postpartum suction evacuation for haemorrhage
D. Second generation endometrial ablation
E. Surgical termination of pregnancy

TOG Article

Shakir F, Diab Y. The perforated uterus. The Obstetrician & Gynaecologist 2013;15:256–261.

Perforation in cases of ERPC for PPH have been reported in 5% of cases.

Perforation for Ashermans syndrome are 0.7–1.8%.

TOP associated with perforation 0.4–0.52% and hysteroscopy for PMB in 0.2–2.0%.

45 What is the most frequently encountered complication of suction evacuation of the uterus for first trimester miscarriage?

A. Haemorrhage

B. Pelvic infection

C. Perforation

D. Retained products of conception

E. Significant Cervical Injury

RCOG Consent Advice 10 Surgical Evacuation of the Uterus for Early Pregnancy Loss

Risk of ERPC:

Perforation 1/200

Haemorrhage 1–2/1000

Pelvic Infection 3/100

Retained Products of Conception 5/100

Cervical tear = rare

46 A 19-year-old woman is to undergo a laparoscopy for pelvic pain. How would you describe the correct technique for entry with the veress needle?

A. Enter below the umbilicus horizontally and then pass the needle at 45° to the skin

B. Enter below the umbilicus transverse plane and then pass the needle at 45° to the skin

C. Enter below the umbilicus vertical to the skin

D. Enter at the base of the umbilicus and pass the needle at ~60° to the skin

E. Enter the base of the umbilicus vertical to the skin

GTG 49 Preventing Entry-Related Gynaecological Laparoscopic Injuries

In most circumstances, the primary incision for laparoscopy should be vertical from the base of the umbilicus (not in the skin below the umbilicus).

Care should be taken not to incise so deeply as to enter the peritoneal cavity.

The Veress needle should be sharp, with a good and tested spring action. A disposable needle is recommended, as it will fulfil these criteria.

The operating table should be horizontal (not in the Trendelenburg tilt) at the start of the procedure.

The abdomen should be palpated to check for any masses and for the position of the aorta before insertion of the Veress needle.

The lower abdominal wall should be stabilised in such a way that the Veress needle can be inserted at right angles to the skin and should be pushed in sufficient enough to penetrate the fascia and the peritoneum. Two audible clicks are usually heard as these layers are penetrated.

47 What is the most common complication of the bottom up single-incision retropubic tape procedure?
A. Bladder perforation
B. De novo urinary urgency
C. Retention
D. Tape erosion
E. Voiding dysfunction

NICE IPG 262 Single-Incision Suburethral Short Tape Insertion for Stress Urinary Incontinence in Women

Four case series reported rates of bladder perforation of up to 3%. In one case series of 40 women, 'vaginal buttonholing' (inadvertent perforation of the vaginal wall) occurred in 5% (2/40) of women.

Tape erosion into the vagina ('tape exposure') was reported in one woman in 1–7%.

De novo voiding dysfunction was reported in up to 5% of women in two separate case series. De novo urgency occurred in up to 16%.

48 You have attempted to perform a direct entry for your laparoscopy and opted to undertake a Palmer's point entry.
Where would you find Palmers point?
A. 1 cm below the left costal margin in the mid-clavicular line
B. 1 cm below the right costal margin in the mid-clavicular line
C. 3 cm below the left costal margin in the mid-axilla
D. 3 cm below the left costal margin in the mid-clavicular line
E. 3 cm inferior to the right intercostal margin

GTG 49 Preventing Entry-Related Gynaecological Laparoscopic Injuries

The preferred point of entry is 3 cm below the left costal margin in the mid-clavicular line (Palmer's point)

49 A laparoscopic hysterectomy has been completed and several port sizes have been used.

When the port is in the midline, what size of port requires closure of the rectus sheath?

A. <5 mm
B. 5 mm
C. 7 mm
D. >10 mm
E. All midline ports

GTG 49 Preventing Entry-Related Gynaecological Laparoscopic Injuries

Any nonmidline port over 7 mm and **any midline port greater than 10 mm requires formal deep sheath closure to avoid the occurrence of port site hernia.**

50 A laparoscopy oophorectomy has been completed and the port sites are about to be closed.

What diameter of nonmidline port site required closure of the rectus sheath?

A. No nonmidline port
B. <5 mm
C. 5 mm
D. >7 mm
E. All midline ports

GTG 49 Preventing Entry-Related Gynaecological Laparoscopic Injuries

Any nonmidline port over 7 mm and any midline port greater than 10 mm requires formal deep sheath closure to avoid the occurrence of port site hernia.

51 A woman is due to undergo an outpatient hysteroscopy and is concerned about pain.

Which hysteroscope is associated with the least discomfort in the outpatient setting?

A. All are the same

B. Flexible Hysteroscope

C. Rigid Hysteroscope 0°

D. Rigid Hysteroscope 15°

E. Rigid Hysteroscope 30°

GTG 59 Best Practice in Outpatient Hysteroscopy

Flexible hysteroscope is associated with less pain during outpatient hysteroscopy compared with rigid hysteroscope.

52 A woman is due to undergo an outpatient hysteroscopic polypectomy using a bipolar resectoscope.

Which distension medium should be used?

A. Glucose 5%

B. Glycine

C. Manitol

D. Normal Saline

E. Purisol

GTG 59 Best Practice in Outpatient Hysteroscopy

Uterine distension with normal saline allows improved image quality and allows outpatient diagnostic hysteroscopy to be completed more quickly compared to uterine distension with carbon dioxide.

Operative outpatient hysteroscopy using **bipolar electrosurgery requires the use of normal saline** to act as both the distension and conducting medium.

53 A woman is due to undergo a routine diagnostic laparoscopy.

According to RCOG data what is the expected incidence of bowel injury during a laparoscopy?

A. <0.1/1000

B. 0.36/1000

C. 3.6/1000

D. 3.6/10,000

E. 3.6/100,000

GTG 49 Preventing Entry-Related Gynaecological Laparoscopic Injuries

A prospective observational study of all gynaecological laparoscopies performed by all grades of staff during a calendar year in a teaching hospital reported bowel damage three times in 836 laparoscopies (3.6/1000).

54 A woman with a stage 3 uterine prolapse is considering a variety of surgical options.

She understands the potential benefits of a mesh repair but is concerned about the risk of mesh erosion.

What is the risk of mesh erosion for a patient undergoing a subtotal hysterectomy with sacrocolpopexy?

A. 4%

B. 7%

C. 14%

D. 18%

E. 24%

NICE IPG284 Sacrocolpopexy with Hysterectomy Using Mesh for Uterine Prolapse Repair

Mesh erosion is the lowest in patients undergoing a subtotal hysterectomy with Sacrocolpopexy (4%) compared to Sacrohysteropexy (8%) and total hysterectomy with Sacrocolpopexy (11%).

55 A woman had a total abdominal hysterectomy in the past using a lower transverse incision.

She has now developed a persistent ovarian cyst and is due to have a laparoscopic bilateral salpingo-oophorectomy.

What will be the incidence of adhesions in the region of the umbilicus in this scenario?

A. 11%

B. 17%

C. 23%

D. 31%

E. 45%

GTG 49 Preventing Entry-Related Gynaecological Laparoscopic Injuries

The rate of adhesion formation at the umbilicus may be up to 50% following midline laparotomy and 23% following low transverse incision.

56 A morbidly obese woman is due to undergo a total laparoscopic hysterectomy for endometrial cancer.

What type of complication is more common compared to traditional open hysterectomy in this situation?

A. Bowel injury

B. Hernia

C. Infection

D. Urinary tract injury

E. Venous thrombosis

NICE IPG 239 Laparoscopic Techniques for Hysterectomy

Clinicians should advise women that there is a higher risk of urinary tract injury and of severe bleeding associated with these procedures, in comparison with open surgery.

57 A woman has been offered a sacrocolpopexy for a vault prolapse. Her friend had a similar operation but developed stress incontinence following the procedure.

What is the incidence of de novo stress incontinence after a sacrocolpopexy?

A. 1–5%

B. 7–12%

C. 14–19%

D. 21–26%

E. 27–32%

NICE IPG284 Sacrocolpopexy with Hysterectomy Using Mesh for Uterine Prolapse Repair

A randomized controlled trial that compared Sacrocolpopexy (mesh) with Sacrospinouscolpopexy (no mesh) reported postoperative de novo stress urinary incontinence in 9% (2/22) of women treated by Sacrocolpopexy (mesh) compared with 33% of women treated by Sacrospinouscolpopexy.

58 A woman presents with a history of dysuria, postmicturition dribble and vaginal discharge.

On examination, a tender mass anteriorly inside the introitus is found. You suspect a urethral diverticulum.

What investigation would you use to diagnose the presence of a urethral diverticulum?

A. Urethroscopy using a 0° endoscope
B. Urethroscopy using a 12° endoscope
C. Urethroscopy using a 30° endoscope
D. Urethroscopy using a 70° endoscope
E. Urodynamics

TOG Article

Archer R, Blackman J, Scott M, Barrington J. Urethral diverticulum. The Obstetrician & Gynaecologist 2015:17:125–129.

Urethroscopy using a 0° endoscope has been the traditional method to investigate and locate a urethra diverticulum. It can detect a mucosal defect in about 70% of patients but, in addition, other pathology such as carcinoma in situ can be ruled out. About 60% of women with a urethral diverticulum would have stress incontinence. Furthermore, 17% of women would develop stress incontinence after excision of the diverticulum. As a result, urodynamics is helpful for baseline assessment of urethral function before surgery but not as helpful in making a diagnosis.

59 A 45-year-old multiparous woman is due to have a hysterectomy for heavy menstrual bleeding. The patient is considering having a subtotal hysterectomy as she has had normal cervical smears history.

When comparing a subtotal hysterectomy to a total hysterectomy, which perioperative complication is reduced?

A. Bowel injury
B. Cyclical vaginal bleeding
C. Intraoperative blood loss
D. Pyrexia
E. Urinary retention

Cochrane Database

Lethaby A, Mukhopadhyay A, Naik R. Total versus subtotal hysterectomy for benign gynaecological conditions. Cochrane Database of Systematic Reviews 2012, Issue 4. Art. No.: CD004993. DOI: 10.1002/14651858.CD004993.pub3.

There is a shorter operating time (11 minutes) and less intraoperative blood loss (57 ml) in patients undergoing subtotal hysterectomies. However, this might have no clinical significance. It is estimated that 13% of patients undergoing subtotal hysterectomies have persistent cyclical vaginal bleeding. There is no difference in the 9 year follow-up of urinary or bowel symptoms. The incidence of postoperative pyrexia is higher in total hysterectomies (8% vs 4%) and urinary retention (OR 0.23 95% CI 0.1–0.8)

60 At the end of a total laparoscopic hysterectomy (in which the woman was placed in a steep Trendelenburg position) you observe that the woman's shoulder brace was placed too laterally.
What type of nerve injury may present in the postoperative period?
A. Femoral nerve injury
B. Lower brachial plexus injury
C. Radial nerve injury
D. Ulnar nerve injury
E. Upper brachial nerve injury

TOG Article

Kuponiyi O, Alleemudder DI, Latunde-Dada A, Eedarapalli P. Nerve injuries associated with gynaecological surgery. The Obstetrician & Gynaecologist 2014;16:29–36.

Brachial plexus injuries occur when shoulder braces are used to provide patient support in the steep Trendelenburg position. The lower brachial plexus nerve roots (C8–T1) are stretched if the brace is positioned too laterally. Hyper-abduction of the arm may result in a lesion of the upper nerve roots of the brachial plexus. This typically occurs when arm boards are extended beyond 90° from the long axis of the operating table. The degree of nerve injury is proportional to blade length.

Antenatal Care

61 A nulliparous woman with a dichorionic diamniotic twin pregnancy presents at 32 weeks gestation with severe pruritis and an
erythematous papular rash on her abdomen with periumbilical
sparing. The most likely diagnosis is:

A. Atopic eruption of pregnancy

B. Eczema

C. Obstetric cholestatsis

D. Pemphigoid gestationis

E. Polymorphic eruption of pregnancy

TOG Article

Maharajan A, Aye C, Ratnavel R, Burova E. Skin eruptions specific
to pregnancy: an overview. The Obstetrician and Gynaecologist 2013;
15:233–240.

Polymorphic eruption of pregnancy occurs in 1:160–1:300 pregnancies, usually presenting in the third trimester. Risk factors are
nulliparity or multiple pregnancy or any other cause of abdominal
overdistension. The condition initially presents with pruritic erythematous papules located within abdominal striae and with periumbilical
sparing.

62 A woman presents at 34 weeks gestation with a sudden onset of
severe headache and altered consciousness following an episode
of vomiting and diarrhoea. What is the most appropriate imaging
technique?

A. Cerebral angiography

B. Computerised tomography (CT scan)

C. Magnetic resonance imaging (MRI scan)

D. Magnetic resonance venography (MRV scan)

E. Skull X-ray

Part 2 MRCOG: Single Best Answer Questions, First Edition.
Andrew Sizer, Chandrika Balachandar, Nibedan Biswas, Richard Foon,
Anthony Griffiths, Sheena Hodgett, Banchhita Sahu and Martyn Underwood.
© 2016 John Wiley & Sons, Ltd. Published 2016 by John Wiley & Sons, Ltd.

Revell K, Morrish P. Headaches in pregnancy. The Obstetrician and Gynaecologist 2014;16:179–184.

Pregnancy is a recognised risk factor for cerebral venous thrombosis (CVT) perhaps as a result of prothrombotic changes and dehydration. Headache is the most common symptom occurring in 80–90% but rarely the only symptom; usually other neurological symptoms are present. The greatest risk period is the third trimester. Computerised tomography is abnormal in only 30% of cases. Magnetic resonance venography (MRV) is the imaging modality of choice.

63 A woman attends for a dating ultrasound scan at 12 weeks gestation. Doppler ultrasound identifies tricuspid regurgitation and a reversed A-wave in the ductus venosus (DV). She is at increased risk of which condition?

    A. Early onset fetal growth restriction (FGR)

    B. Early onset pre-eclampsia

    C. Fetal anaemia

    D. Fetal aneuploidy

    E. Late onset pre-eclampsia

TOG Article

Mone F, McAuliffe F, Ong S. The clinical application of Doppler ultrasound in obstetrics. The Obstetrician and Gynaecologist 2015;17:13–19.

A role for tricuspid regurgitation and DV is in first trimester screening with a significant association between the presence of tricuspid regurgitation and of a reversed A-wave in the DV between 11 and 13 + 6 weeks of gestation and the presence of fetal aneuploidy or congenital cardiac defects.

64 A woman is referred by the community midwife with suspected small for dates pregnancy at 33 weeks gestation. Ultrasound assessment confirms a small for gestation (SGA) fetus with reduced liquor volume and reversed end diastolic flow on umbilical artery (UA) Doppler. Cardiotocograph (CTG) is normal. What is the most appropriate management?

    A. Antenatal steroids and delivery within 1 week

    B. Elective delivery at 37 weeks gestation

    C. Immediate delivery by caesarean section

    D. Repeat Doppler ultrasound in 1 week

    E. Repeat ultrasound growth assessment in 2 weeks

TOG Article

Mone F, McAuliffe F, Ong S. The clinical application of Doppler ultrasound in obstetrics. The Obstetrician and Gynaecologist 2015; 17:13–19.

An abnormal UA Doppler waveform (absent or reversed end-diastolic flow) has been demonstrated to predict fetal compromise. This pattern appears to be present 12 days preceding acute fetal deterioration.

65 What proportion of pre-eclampsia can be predicted by risk assessment from maternal history alone in the first trimester of pregnancy?
A. 10–20%
B. 20–30%
C. 30–40%
D. 40–50%
E. 50–60%

TOG Article

Mone F, McAuliffe F. Low-dose aspirin and calcium supplementation for the prevention of pre-eclampsia. The Obstetrician and Gynaecologist 2014;16:245–250.

Maternal history at the booking visit alone as a form of first trimester risk assessment for pre-eclampsia can predict 47% of cases of both early and late onset pre-eclampsia with a false positive rate of 10%.

66 When aspirin is used to reduce risk of pre-eclampsia in woman at high risk, at what gestation should it be commenced for maximum efficacy?
A. Before 12 weeks
B. Before 16 weeks
C. Before 20 weeks
D. Before 24 weeks
E. Before 28 weeks

TOG Article

Mone F, McAuliffe F. Low-dose aspirin and calcium supplementation for the prevention of pre-eclampsia. The Obstetrician and Gynaecologist 2014;16:245–250.

The maximum potential effect in terms of adverse perinatal outcome is seen when aspirin is commenced before 16 weeks of gestation.

67 When calcium supplementation is used to reduce the risk of pre-eclampsia in women at high risk, at what gestation should it be commenced?

A. 12 weeks

B. 16 weeks

C. 20 weeks

D. 24 weeks

E. 28 weeks

TOG Article

Mone F, McAuliffe F. Low-dose aspirin and calcium supplementation for the prevention of pre-eclampsia. The Obstetrician and Gynaecologist 2014;16:245–250.

The World Health Organisation (WHO) advises calcium supplements at a dosage of 1.5–2 g per day from 20 weeks gestation in populations where calcium intake is low, to prevent the onset of pre-eclampsia, especially among women who are at high risk. Twenty weeks is the gestation at which most evidence exists and when maternal levels begin to fall.

68 What proportion of pregnant women in the United Kingdom is estimated to take the recommended dose of periconceptual folic acid supplementation?

A. less than 5%

B. 5–10%

C. 10–20%

D. 20–50%

E. 50–70%

TOG Article

Duckworth S, Mistry H, Chappell L. Vitamin supplementation in pregnancy. The Obstetrician and Gynaecologist 2012;14:175–178.

Despite NICE guidance recommending folic acid supplementation, a recent systematic review estimated the use of periconceptional folic acid in the United Kingdom to be 21–48%.

69 What is the incidence of red cell antibodies in pregnancy?

A. 1 in 500

B. 1 in 300

C. 1 in 160

D. 1 in 80

E. 1 in 40

GTG 65 The Management of Women with Red Cell Antibodies During Pregnancy

What is the incidence of red cell antibodies in pregnancy?

In a population study conducted in the Netherlands, the prevalence of positive antibody screens was 1:80.

70 In the presence of anti-c red cell antibodies in pregnancy, which additional red cell antibody increases the risk of fetal anaemia?

A. Anti-D

B. Anti-e

C. Anti-E

D. Anti-Fy^a

E. Anti-K

GTG 65 The Management of Women with Red Cell Antibodies During Pregnancy

The presence of anti-E potentiates the severity of fetal anaemia due to anti-c antibodies; so, unless the fetus has only one of these antigens, referral at lower levels/titres is indicated.

71 A woman attends the antenatal clinic following a scan at 36 weeks gestation in her fourth pregnancy, which identifies an anterior placenta previa. She has had three previous caesarean births. What is the risk of placenta accreta?

A. 3%

B. 11%

C. 40%

D. 61%

E. 67%

TOG Article

Dahlke J, Mendez-Figueroa H, Wenstrom K. Counselling women about the risks of caesarean delivery in future pregnancies. The Obstetrician and Gynaecologist 2014;16:239–244.

In a prospective study of over 30,000 women undergoing elective caesarean delivery (CD), women with placenta previa had a risk of placenta accreta in 3%, 11%, 40%, 61% and 67% for first, second, third, fourth and fifth or more CDs.

72 What proportion of pregnant women in paid employment require time off work due to nausea and vomiting of pregnancy (NVP)?
A. 10%
B. 20%
C. 30%
D. 40%
E. 50%

TOG Article

Gadsby R, Barnie-Adshead T. Severe nausea and vomiting of pregnancy: should it be treated with appropriate pharmacotherapy? The Obstetrician and Gynaecologist 2011;13:107–111.

Approximately 30% of pregnant working women need time off from paid employment because of NVP.

73 What is the incidence of acute appendicitis in pregnancy?
A. 1 in 400 to 1 in 800
B. 1 in 800 to 1 in 1500
C. 1 in 1500 to 1 in 2000
D. 1 in 2000 to 1 in 2500
E. 1 in 3000

TOG Article

Weston P, Moroz P. Appendicitis in pregnancy: how to manage and whether to deliver. The Obstetrician and Gynaecologist 2015;17:105–110.

In developed countries, acute appendicitis is suspected in 1 in 800 pregnancies and confirmed in 1 in 800 to 1 in 1500. Its incidence is most common in the second trimester.

74 A 21-year-old woman is admitted at 22 weeks gestation in her first pregnancy with suspected appendicitis. She has a low grade pyrexia with a leucocytosis and a mildly elevated C reactive protein level. Abdominal ultrasound is inconclusive. What imaging technique is the most appropriate subsequent investigation?
A. Abdominal X-ray
B. Computed tomography (CT) scan of the abdomen
C. Magnetic resonance imaging (MRI) scan of the abdomen
D. Repeat abdominal ultrasound in 24 hours
E. Transvaginal ultrasound scan of the pelvis

TOG Article

Weston P, Moroz P. Appendicitis in pregnancy: how to manage and whether to deliver. The Obstetrician and Gynaecologist 2015;17:105–110.

Evaluation of MRI in pregnant women with suspected appendicitis confers a sensitivity of 91% and a specificity of 98%. The American College of Radiology dictates that MRI should be used in cases where ultrasound is inconclusive for appendicitis in pregnancy.

75 What is the risk of serious neonatal infection associated with prelabour rupture of membranes (PROM) at term?

A. 0.5%

B. 1%

C. 1.5%

D. 2%

E. 2.5%

NICE CG 190 Intrapartum Care: Care of Healthy Women and Their Babies During Childbirth

Advise women presenting with PROM at term that the risk of serious neonatal infection is 1%, rather than 0.5% for women with intact membranes.

76 A women in her first trimester scores more than 3 in the 2-item Generalized Anxiety Disorder scale (GAD-2) used to identify anxiety disorders in pregnancy.

What is the best plan of care?

A. Further assess using the GAD-10 scale

B. Further assess using the GAD-7 scale

C. Reassure

D. Repeat the GAD-2 scale in 4 weeks

E. Repeat the GAD-2 scale in second trimester

NICE CG 192 Antenatal and Postnatal Mental Health

If a woman scores 3 or more on the GAD-2 scale, consider:

Using the GAD-7 scale for further assessment or

Refer the woman to her GP or, if a severe mental health problem is suspected, to a mental health professional.

77 Women suffer from various anxieties in pregnancy.
What is tokophobia?
A. Fear of baby dying in utero
B. Fear of extreme pain
C. Extreme fear of childbirth
D. Fear of heights
E. Fear of spiders

NICE CG 192 Antenatal and Postnatal Mental Health

For a woman with tokophobia (an extreme fear of childbirth), offer an opportunity to discuss her fears with a health-care professional with expertise in providing perinatal mental health support.

78 What vitamin should women be advised to be taken throughout pregnancy and also while breastfeeding?
A. Folic acid
B. Vitamin A
C. Vitamin C
D. Vitamin D
E. Vitamin K

NICE CG 62 Antenatal Care

All women should be informed at the booking appointment about the importance of their own and their baby's health of maintaining adequate vitamin D stores during pregnancy and while breastfeeding. In order to achieve this, women should be advised to take a vitamin D supplement (10 micrograms of vitamin D per day)

79 An 18-year-old woman books into the antenatal clinic at 12 weeks of gestation. She is fit and well but is noted to have an increased body mass index (BMI) but no other risk factors for diabetes.
What BMI and above should she be offered screening for diabetes?
A. 25
B. 30
C. 35
D. 38
E. 40

Screening for gestational diabetes using risk factors is recommended in a healthy population. At the booking appointment, the following risk factors for gestational diabetes should be determined:

- BMI above 30 kg/m²
- Previous macrosomic baby weighing 4.5 kg or above
- Previous gestational diabetes
- Family history of diabetes (first-degree relative with diabetes)
- Family origin with a high prevalence of diabetes: South Asian (specifically women whose country of family origin is India, Pakistan or Bangladesh) black Caribbean, middle eastern (specifically women whose country of family origin is Saudi Arabia, United Arab Emirates, Iraq, Jordan, Syria, Oman, Qatar, Kuwait, Lebanon or Egypt).

Women with any **one** of these risk factors should be offered testing for gestational diabetes

80 An anxious woman attends the antenatal clinic. She is planning an afternoon picnic and has a list of her favourite foods including UHT milk, cottage cheese sandwiches, vegetable pate, lambs kidneys and baked oily fish.

Which of these food products is not recommended in pregnancy due to the risk of listeriosis?

A. Cottage cheese
B. Lamb's kidneys
C. Oily fish
D. UHT milk
E. **Vegetable pate**

NICE CG 62 Antenatal Care

Pregnant women should be offered information on how to reduce the risk of listeriosis by:

Drinking only pasteurised or UHT milk

Not eating ripened soft cheese such as Camembert, Brie and blue-veined cheese (there is no risk with hard cheeses, such as Cheddar, or cottage cheese, and processed cheese).

Not eating pâté (of any sort, including vegetable)

Not eating uncooked or undercooked ready-prepared meals.

81 A woman is advised to avoid drinking all alcohol in pregnancy but she declines. She enjoys wine but no more than 250 ml per week. She is keen to understand the safe limits of alcohol intake.

What is acceptable with regard to alcohol intake during pregnancy?

A. 1–2 UK Units per week

B. 3–4 UK Units per week

C. 5–6 UK Units per week

D. 7–8 UK Units per week

E. 9–10 UK Units per week

NICE CG 62 Antenatal Care

If women choose to drink alcohol during pregnancy they should be advised to drink no more than 1 to 2 UK units once or twice a week (1 unit equals half a pint of ordinary strength lager or beer, or one shot [25 ml] of spirits. One small [125 ml] glass of wine is equal to 1.5 UK units). Although there is uncertainty regarding a safe level of alcohol consumption in pregnancy, at this low level there is no evidence of harm to the unborn baby.

82 A women presents with vaginal candidiasis at 23 week pregnancy. What treatment should you offer her?

A. One stat treatment of live yogurt

B. One stat treatment of topical imidazole

C. One week course of oral Ketoconazole

D. One week course of oral nystatin

E. One week course of topical imidazole

NICE CG 62 Antenatal Care

A 1-week course of a topical imidazole is an effective treatment and should be considered for vaginal candidiasis infections in pregnant women. The effectiveness and safety of oral treatments for vaginal candidiasis in pregnancy are uncertain and these treatments should not be offered.

83 You have been asked to review a full blood test results of a woman at 28 weeks of gestation. At what threshold level of haemoglobin concentration would you define anaemia at this gestation?

A. 90 g/l

B. 95 g/l

C. 100 g/l

D. 105 g/l

E. 110 g/l

NICE CG 62 Antenatal Care

Haemoglobin levels outside the normal UK range for pregnancy (that is, 11 g/dl at first contact and 10.5 g/dl at 28 weeks) should be investigated and iron supplementation considered if indicated.

Pregnant women should be offered screening for anaemia. Screening should take place early in pregnancy (at the booking appointment) and at 28 weeks when other blood screening tests are being performed. This allows enough time for treatment if anaemia is detected.

84 A pregnant woman undergoes a routine anomaly ultrasound scan at 18 weeks of gestation. No ultrasound soft markers are present.

At what nuchal translucency measurement is it recommended to refer the woman to fetal medicine services?

A. 2 mm+

B. 3 mm+

C. 4 mm+

D. 5 mm+

E. 6 mm+

NICE CG 62 Antenatal Care

The presence of an isolated soft marker, with the exception of increased nuchal fold, on the routine anomaly scan, should not be used to adjust the a priori risk for Down's syndrome. The presence of an increased nuchal fold (6 mm or above) or two or more soft markers on the routine anomaly scan should prompt the offer of a referral to a fetal medicine specialist or an appropriate health-care professional with a special interest in fetal medicine.

85 A woman is noted to have a low-lying placenta at her 20-week anomaly scan. At what gestational age should you arrange the next scan to assess placental localisation?

A. 28 weeks

B. 30 weeks

C. 32 weeks

D. 34 weeks

E. 36 weeks

NICE CG 62 Antenatal Care

Because most low-lying placentas detected at the routine anomaly scan would have resolved by the time the baby is born, only a woman whose placenta extends over the internal cervical os should be offered another transabdominal scan at 32 weeks. If the transabdominal scan is unclear, a transvaginal scan should be offered.

86 A woman declines an induction of labour at 42 weeks of gestation, the indication being 'post-dates'. What is the recommended for assessment of 'fetal wellbeing' in this situation?
A. CTG three times a day
B. CTG twice daily and weekly Doppler assessment of the umbilical arteries blood flow
C. **CTG twice weekly with an assessment of deepest vertical pool of liquor on ultrasound**
D. CTG weekly with Doppler of the umbilical arteries
E. Weekly Doppler assessment of the umbilical arteries blood flow only

NICE CG 62 Antenatal Care
From 42 weeks, women who decline induction of labour should be offered increased antenatal monitoring consisting of at least twice-weekly cardiotocography and ultrasound estimation of maximum amniotic pool depth

87 A woman at 36 weeks of gestation presents with an uncomplicated breech presentation and consents to undergo an external cephalic version (ECV) after consultation. Unfortunately, due to logistics, this service will not be available when she is 37 weeks.
What management is most appropriate?
A. Elective caesarean section at 37 weeks
B. Elective caesarean section at 38 weeks
C. **ECV at 36 weeks**
D. ECV at 38 weeks
E. Induction of labour 37 weeks to avoid potential cord prolapse

NICE CG 62 Antenatal Care
All women who have an uncomplicated singleton breech pregnancy at 36 weeks should be offered external cephalic version. Exceptions include women in labour and women with a uterine scar or abnormality, fetal compromise, ruptured membranes, vaginal bleeding and medical conditions. Where it is not possible to schedule an appointment for ECV at 37 weeks, it should be scheduled at 36 weeks.

88 A pregnant woman at 34 weeks gestation is complaining of severe chronic sleep problem.

What would be the most appropriate pharmacological intervention?

A. Diazepam

B. Fluoxetine

C. Imipramine

D. Lithium

E. **Promethazine**

NICE CG 192 Antenatal and Postnatal Mental Health

Advice pregnant women who have a sleep problem about sleep hygiene (including having a healthy bedtime routine, avoiding caffeine and reducing activity before sleep). For women with a severe or chronic sleep problem, consider promethazine.

89 A woman undergoes a successful external cephalic version at 37 weeks gestation.

What is the chance of spontaneous reversion to breech?

A. **<5%**

B. 6–8%

C. 10–12%

D. 14–16%

E. 18–20%

GTG 20a External Cephalic Version and Reducing the Incidence of Breech Presentation

Spontaneous reversion to breech presentation after successful ECV occurs in less than 5%.

90 Which tocolytic agent has been proven to increase the success of an ECV?

A. Glyceryl trinitrate (GTN) patch

B. Glyceryl trinitrate (GTN) sublingually

C. Magnesium sulphate infusion

D. Nifedipine

E. **Terbutaline**

GTG 20a External Cephalic Version and Reducing the Incidence of Breech Presentation

The use of tocolysis should be considered where an initial attempt at ECV without tocolysis has failed.

The success rate of ECV is increased by the use of tocolysis. This has been proven with ritodrine, salbutamol and terbutaline but not with glyceryl trinitrate (GTN) as a patch, or sublingually, or with nifedipine. Intravenous and subcutaneous routes can be used. Data on those women who have benefitted most are contradictory. Tocolysis is also beneficial where an initial attempt without it has failed and can be attempted immediately. However, this policy has not been compared to tocolysis for all. A simple protocol is to offer a slow intravenous or subcutaneous bolus of salbutamol or terbutaline either routinely or if an initial ECV attempt has failed.

91 A Gravida 3, Para 2 (both full term normal deliveries) is diagnosed with breech presentation at 35 + 1 weeks of gestation and is keen to have an external cephalic version.
At what gestation is external cephalic version recommended for this mother?
A. 35 weeks
B. 36 weeks
C. 37 weeks
D. 38 weeks
E. 39 weeks

GTG 20a External Cephalic Version and Reducing the Incidence of Breech Presentation

ECV should be offered from 36 weeks in nulliparous women and from 37 weeks in multiparous women.

92 A primigravida aged 26 is admitted with threatened preterm labour at 30 weeks and seeks counselling with regards to antenatal corticosteroids.
What are the three recognised fetal benefits associated with antenatal corticosteroid administration in the case of premature delivery?
A. Reduced respiratory distress syndrome, reduced incidence of hypoglycemia, reduced neonatal death rates
B. Reduced respiratory distress syndrome, reduced VII nerve damage, reduced incidence of hypoglycemia
C. Reduced respiratory distress syndrome, reduce incidence of pneumothorax formation, reduced retinal disease of prematurity
D. Reduced respiratory distress syndrome, reduced intraventricular haemorrhage reduced neonatal death rate
E. Reduced respiratory distress syndrome, reduced intraventricular haemorrhage reduced necrotising enterocolitis rates

GTG 7 Antenatal Corticosteroids to Reduce Neonatal Morbidity and Mortality

The Cochrane reviewed 21 good quality randomised controlled studies and found there was a reduction in:

- Neonatal deaths 31% (95% CI 19–42%)
- Reduced respiratory distress syndrome 44% (95% CI 31–57%)
- Reduced intraventricular haemorrhage 46% (95% CI 31–67%).

Antenatal corticosteroid use is also associated with:

- A reduction in necrotising enterocolitis
- Respiratory support
- Intensive care admissions
- Systemic infections in the first 48 hours of life compared with no treatment or treatment with placebo.

93 A woman who had a previous second trimester miscarriage is currently undergoing a serial ultrasound assessment of cervical length. With what cervical ultrasound feature would cervical cerlage be recommended?

A. **Cervical length less than 25 mm before 24 weeks of gestation**

B. Cervical length less than 30 mm before 24 weeks of gestation

C. Cervical length less than 45 mm before 24 weeks of gestation

D. Funneling of the internal os and a cervical length less than 30 mm

E. Funneling of the internal os before 24 weeks of gestation

GTG 60 Cervical Cerclage

Women with a history of one or more spontaneous mid-trimester losses or preterm births who are undergoing transvaginal sonographic surveillance of cervical length should be offered an ultrasound indicated cerclage if the cervix is 25 mm or less and before 24 weeks of gestation. An ultrasound-indicated cerclage is not recommended for funneling of the cervix (dilatation of the internal os on ultrasound) in the absence of cervical shortening to 25 mm or less.

94 A woman at 32 weeks gestation is admitted with severe falciparum malaria. What is the pharmacological treatment of choice?

A. **Artesunate**

B. Chloroquine

C. Primaquine

D. Quinine

E. Quinine and glucose infusion

GTG 54b The Diagnosis and Treatment of Malaria in Pregnancy

Intravenous artesunate is the treatment of choice for severe falciparum malaria. Use intravenous quinine if artesunate is not available.

Use quinine and clindamycin to treat uncomplicated *P. falciparum* (or mixed, such as *P. falciparum* and *P. vivax*).

Use chloroquine to treat *P. vivax*, *P. ovale* or *P. malariae*.

Primaquine should not be used in pregnancy.

95 A woman who is in the second trimester of pregnancy is planning to travel to an area endemic for chloroquine-resistant malaria. What would you recommend as the drug of choice for prophylaxis?

A. Artusenate

B. Chloroquine

C. Mefloquine

D. Nonpharmacological preventative agents

E. Quinine

GTG 54b The Diagnosis and Treatment of Malaria in Pregnancy

Mefloquine (5 mg/kg once a week) is the recommended drug of choice for prophylaxis in the second and third trimesters for chloroquine-resistant areas. With very few areas in the world free from chloroquine resistance, mefloquine is essentially the only drug considered safe for prophylaxis in pregnant travellers.

96 The velocimetry measurement of blood vessels can be used to improve perinatal outcomes in high-risk pregnancies. Which vessel is assessed?

A. Middle cerebral artery

B. Umbilical artery

C. Umbilical vein

D. Uterine artery

E. Uterine vein

TOG Article

Mone F, McAuliffe FM, Ong S. The clinical application of Doppler ultrasound in obstetrics. The Obstetrician & Gynaecologist 2015;17:13–19.

Umbilical artery Doppler velocimetry has been shown to improve perinatal outcome in high-risk pregnancies, through a meta-analysis of randomised controlled trials.

97 A gravida 2 Para 0 + 1 molar pregnancy is diagnosed with Rhesus isoimmunisation.

Doppler assessment of which vessel is used to monitor fetal anaemia during pregnancy

A. Middle cerebral artery

B. Umbilical artery

C. Umbilical vein

D. Uterine artery

E. Uterine vein

TOG Article

Mone F, McAuliffe FM, Ong S. The clinical application of Doppler ultrasound in obstetrics. The Obstetrician & Gynaecologist 2015;17:13–19.

The role of the MCA Doppler in the management of FGR is less clear than its role in fetal anaemia when the peak systolic velocity (PSV) measurement can be used to assess pregnancies at risk of fetal anaemia, for example, Rhesus isoimmunisation. In this instance, a PSV value greater than 1.5 multiples of the median (MoM) is predictive of fetal anaemia.

98 A woman presents at 26 + 5 weeks of gestation in her first pregnant with reduced fetal movements.

What is the most appropriate initial investigation to carry out?

A. Biophysical profile

B. CTG

C. Doppler auscultation

D. Ultrasound biometry

E. Uterine artery Doppler

GTG 57 Reduced Fetal Movements

If a woman presents with |reduced fetal movements (RFM) between 24 + 0 and 28 + 0 weeks of gestation, the presence of a fetal heartbeat should be confirmed by auscultation with a Doppler handheld device.

There are no studies looking at the outcome of women who present with RFM between 24 + 0 and 28 + 0 weeks of gestation. The fetal heartbeat should be confirmed to check fetal viability. History must include a comprehensive stillbirth risk evaluation, including a review of the presence of other risk factors associated with an increased risk of stillbirth. Clinicians should be aware that placental insufficiency may present at this gestation. There is no evidence to recommend the routine use of CTG surveillance in this group. If there is clinical suspicion of FGR, consideration should be given to the need for ultrasound assessment. There is no evidence on which to recommend the routine use of ultrasound assessment in this group.

99 Domestic violence during pregnancy increases the risk of maternal mortality.

What is the increase in homicide risk when there is domestic violence during pregnancy?

A. two fold

B. three fold

C. four fold

D. five fold

E. six fold

TOG Article

Gottlieb AS. Domestic violence: a clinical guide for women's health care providers. The Obstetrician & Gynaecologist 2012;14:197–202.

Abuse during pregnancy is also a marker for risk of death from domestic violence, conferring a threefold increase in homicide risk and making domestic homicide one of the leading causes of maternal mortality.

100 A woman who is 28 weeks pregnant in her first pregnancy attends the antenatal clinic. She has no medical problems, but on routine questioning, she discloses domestic abuse. She insists that this information has not been disclosed to anyone else.

What is the first action that should be undertaken?

A. Contact the Police

B. Contact the Independent Domestic Violence Advocate (IDVA) for advice

C. Document the consultation fully in the hand-held record

D. Perform a safety assessment

E. Persuade the woman to leave her partner and seek refuge in a shelter

TOG Article

Gottlieb AS. Domestic violence: a clinical guide for women's health care providers. The Obstetrician & Gynaecologist 2012; 14:197–202.

The clinician should then perform a brief safety assessment to establish the severity of the situation. The use of weapons and homicidal threats increase a woman's risk of being murdered.

Therefore, some important questions to ask are:

Does your abuser have a weapon?

Has he made threats to kill you?

Do you feel safe to go home now?

101 A course of antenatal corticosteroids is associated with a significant reduction in neonatal morbidity and mortality in women who are at risk of preterm birth.
What is the reduction in risk of intraventricular haemorrhage?
A. 5%
B. 12%
C. 26%
D. 46%
E. 68%

GTG 7 Antenatal Corticosteroids to Reduce Neonatal Morbidity and Mortality

A Cochrane review of 21 studies (3885 women and 4269 infants) showed that treatment of women at risk of preterm birth with a single course of antenatal corticosteroids reduced the risk of neonatal death by 31% (95% CI 19–42%), RDS by 44% (95% CI 31–57%) and intraventricular haemorrhage by 46% (95% CI 31–67%).

102 What proportion of twin pregnancies have monochorionic placentation?
A. 10%
B. 25%
C. 33%
D. 50%
E. 67%

GTG 51 Management of Monochorionic Twin Pregnancy

A monochorionic twin pregnancy is one in which both babies are dependent on a single, shared placenta.

Around one-third of twin pregnancies in the United Kingdom have monochorionic placentas.

103 What proportion of monchorionic twin pregnancies are complicated by twin to twin transfusion syndrome (TTTS)?
A. 1–2%
B. 10–15%
C. 25–30%
D. 50–60%
E. 70–80%

GTG 51 Management of Monochorionic Twin Pregnancy

TTTS complicates 10–15% of MC pregnancies; the placentas are more likely to have unidirectional artery–vein anastomoses and less likely to have bidirectional artery–artery anastomoses.

104 A woman with a monchorionic diamniotic twin pregnancy at 25 weeks gestation is assessed at the regional fetal medicine service. She is found to have severe TTTS (Quintero stage III).

What is the optimal treatment?

A. Amnioreduction

B. Fetoscopic laser ablation

C. Septostomy

D. Termination of the donor twin

E. Termination of the entire pregnancy

GTG 51 Management of Monochorionic Twin Pregnancy

Severe TTTS presenting before 26 weeks of gestation should be treated by laser ablation rather than by amnioreduction or septostomy.

Some women request termination of pregnancy when severe TTTS is diagnosed and this should be discussed as an option. Another option is to offer selective termination of pregnancy using bipolar diathermy of one of the umbilical cords, which will result in the inevitable sacrifice of that baby. This may be appropriate if there is severe hydrops fetalis in the recipient or evidence of cerebral damage in either twin.

105 A 30-year-old primagravida with a BMI of 28 is seen in the antenatal clinic at 36 weeks gestation following referral from the community midwife with suspected 'large-for dates'.

An ultrasound scan is arranged, which confirms the fetus to be large for gestational age.

An oral glucose tolerance test is arranged a few days later, which is normal.

What is the correct management?

A. Elective caesarean section at 38 weeks

B. Elective caesarean section at 39 weeks

C. Induction of labour at 37 weeks

D. Induction of labour at 40 weeks

E. Induction of labour at 40 weeks + 10 days

TOG Article

Aye SS, MillerV, Saxena S, Farhan M. Management of large-for-gestational-age pregnancy in non-diabetic women. The Obstetrician & Gynaecologist, 2010;12:250–256.

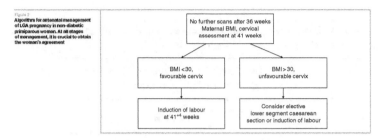

Figure 2
Algorithm for antenatal management of LGA pregnancy in non-diabetic primiparous woman. At all stages of management, it is crucial to obtain the woman's agreement

No further scans after 36 weeks
Maternal BMI, cervical assessment at 41 weeks

BMI <30, favourable cervix — Induction of labour at 41^{+4} weeks

BMI >30, unfavourable cervix — Consider elective lower segment caesarean section or induction of labour

106 In the United Kingdom, the perinatal mortality rate is approximately 7 per 1000 births.
What is the perinatal mortality rate in monoamniotic twin pregnancies?
A. 10–30 per 1000
B. 30–70 per 1000
C. 100–300 per 1000
D. 300–700 per 1000
E. 700–900 per 1000

TOG Article

Dias T, Thilaganathan B, Bhide A. Monoamniotic twin pregnancy. The Obstetrician & Gynaecologist 2012;14:71–78.

Perinatal mortality of monoamniotic twins has been reported to be as high as 30–70%.

107 A healthy 35-year-old woman attends the antenatal clinic at 37 weeks gestation in her third pregnancy. She has had two previous caesarean sections for breech presentation, but the current pregnancy has a cephalic presentation and she would like to have a vaginal birth after caesarean (VBAC).
What would be the risk of uterine rupture if she labours with such a history?
A. 0.4–0.5%
B. 0.7–0.9%
C. 0.9–1.8%
D. 2.5–3.1%
E. 4.8–6.7%

TOG Article

Dahlke JD, Mendez-Figueroa H, Wenstrom KD. Counselling women about the risks of caesarean delivery in future pregnancies. The Obstetrician & Gynaecologist 2014;16:239–244.

Table 3. Comparison of maternal and neonatal risks between repeat caesarean and trial of labour after caesarean[12]

	Repeat caesarean (%)	Trial of labour after caesarean (%)	
Maternal risks		After 1 caesarean	After 2 caesareans
Uterine rupture	0.4–0.5	0.7–0.9	0.9–1.8
Hysterectomy	0–0.4	0.2–0.5	0.6
Blood transfusion	1–1.4	0.7–1.7	3.2
Endometritis	1.5–2.1	2.9	3.1
Operative injury	0.4–0.6	0.4	0.4
Maternal death	0.02–0.04	0.02	0
Neonatal risks		Trial of labour after caesarean (%)	
Stillbirth			
37–38 weeks	0.08	0.38	
≥39 weeks	0.01	0.16	
Neonatal death	0.05	0.08	
Hypoxic ischaemic encephalopathy	0–0.013	0.08	
Respiratory morbidity	1–5	0.1–1.8	
Transient tachypnoea	6.2	3.5	
Hyperbilirubinemia	5.8	2.2	

108 A 41-year-old woman with a BMI of 36 kg/m², but otherwise healthy, attends the antenatal clinic at 14 weeks gestation and is found to have a dichorionic diamniotic twin pregnancy.

What supplementation would you advise to reduce her risk of developing pre-eclampsia?

A. Aspirin 75 mg daily until 28 weeks

B. Aspirin 75 mg daily until term

C. Aspirin 150 mg daily until 34 weeks

D. Calcium 1 mg daily until 20 weeks

E. Calcium 10 mg daily until term

TOG Article

Mone F, McAuliffe FM. Low-dose aspirin and calcium supplementation for the prevention of pre-eclampsia. The Obstetrician & Gynaecologist 2014;16:245–250.

If a patient has two moderate risk factors or one major risk factor, clinicians are advised to prescribe 75 mg of aspirin from 12 weeks of gestation until delivery. These risk factors are summarised in Table 2.

Table 2. Indications for low-dose aspirin use in pregnancy for pre-eclampsia prevention

High risk	Moderate risk
Hypertensive disease in previous pregnancy	Primigravida
Chronic kidney disease	Age >40 years
Auto immune disease e.g. anti-phospholipid syndrome	Pregnancy interval >10 years
Diabetes mellitus	Family history pre-eclampsia
Chronic hypertension	Multiple pregnancy
	BMI >35 kg/m² at booking

109 During pregnancy, how much calcium is accumulated by the fetus?
   A. 1–2 g
   B. 10–15 g
   C. **25–30 g**
   D. 70–100 g
   E. 150–200 g

TOG Article

Mone F, McAuliffe FM. Low-dose aspirin and calcium supplementation for the prevention of pre-eclampsia. The Obstetrician & Gynaecologist 2014;16:245–250.

In pregnancy, serum levels of calcium tend to fall due to active transport across the placenta to the fetus, which can accumulate up to 25–30 g over the course of the pregnancy, notably in the third trimester.

110 A 26-year-old primagravida with a singleton pregnancy at 23 weeks gestation attends for an ultrasound scan following a small amount of vaginal bleeding.

It is noted that the cervical length is 21 mm.

What is the appropriate management?

A. Antenatal corticosteroids

B. Expectant management

C. Insertion of a McDonald suture

D. Insertion of a Shirodkar suture

E. Tocolytic therapy

GTG 60 Cervical Cerclage

The insertion of an ultrasound-indicated cerclage is not recommended in women without a history of spontaneous preterm delivery or second-trimester loss who have an incidentally identified short cervix of 25 mm or less.

111 Which protein is the most important biomarker for the detection of PPROM (Preterm Prelabour Rupture of Membranes)?

A. Nitrazine

B. Placental alkaline phosphatase

C. Placental Alpha Microglobulin-1 (PAMG-1)

D. Placental vasopressinase

E. Pregnancy-associated plasma protein A

Detection of Placental Alpha Microglobulin-1 (PAMG-1) with a Monoclonal Antibody Is the Basis of the *Aminsure* Test

112 What is the usual method of diagnosing placental abruption?

A. Clinical diagnosis

B. D-dimer level

C. Kleihauer test

D. Transabdominal ultrasound

E. Transvaginal ultrasound

GTG 63 Antepartum Haemorrhage

Placental abruption is a clinical diagnosis and there are no sensitive or reliable diagnostic tests available. Ultrasound has limited sensitivity in the identification of retroplacental haemorrhage.

The Kleihauer test is not a sensitive test for diagnosing abruption.

113 A primigravida with a low-risk pregnancy is admitted at 30 weeks with an antepartum haemorrhage (APH). A diagnosis of placental abruption has been made. The bleeding settled with conservative management and she is discharged home.

What is the most appropriate plan for her further antenatal care?

A. Advise continued hospital stay

B. Reassure and continue with midwife-led care and arrange for induction of labour at term + 10 days

C. Reassure and continue with midwife-led care as the bleeding has settled

D. Reclassify as 'high risk' and arrange consultant-led care

E. Reclassify as 'high risk', arrange consultant-led care with serial ultrasound for fetal growth

GTG 63 Antepartum Haemorrhage

Women with APH are at increased risk of adverse perinatal outcome, growth restriction, in particular, and increased fetal surveillance is recommended.

114 A 35-year-old primigravida is seen in the antenatal clinic for booking. She had been diagnosed with breast cancer at the age of 32 and received adjuvant chemotherapy with doxorubicin following surgery.

What is the most appropriate management?

A. Advise termination of pregnancy

B. Arrange echocardiography to detect risk of cardiomyopathy

C. Arrange outpatient ECG and 24 hour cardiac monitoring to detect risk of cardiomyopathy

D. Make a referral to the Oncologist

E. Reassure and plan consultant led antenatal care

GTG 12 Pregnancy and Breast Cancer

ECG and 24 hour cardiac monitoring does not detect cardiomyopathy. Anthracylines such as doxorubicin and epirubicin are cardiotoxic and cause cumulative dose-dependent left ventricular dysfunction. Risk of cardiomyopathy is best diagnosed with echocardiography through resting left ventricular ejection fraction or echocardiographic fractional shortening.

115 You receive a telephone call from a community midwife. A 22-year- old primigravida, currently 15 weeks pregnant, has developed chickenpox and the rash had developed 72 hours ago.

The mother is very anxious and the midwife requests advice with regard to further management.

What would you advise?

A. To inform the mother about the risk of fetal varicella syndrome and advice termination of pregnancy once she overcomes the infective stage

B. To reassure the mother and a course of Aciclovir to be obtained from the General Practitioner

C. To reassure the mother and arrange for VZIG administration from the General Practitioner

D. To reassure the mother that the risk of spontaneous miscarriage is not increased and arrange referral to a fetal medicine specialist for further advice and a detailed ultrasound

E. To reassure the mother that the risk of spontaneous miscarriage is not increased and arrange referral to a fetal medicine specialist for amniocentesis to rule out Fetal Varicella Syndrome

GTG 13 Chickenpox in Pregnancy

Aciclovir should be used cautiously before 20 weeks and is only effective if commenced within 24 hours of onset of the rash. VZIG is not effective for active infection and is only used if the mother is not immune and has had a significant exposure for prevention. Amniocentesis is not routinely advised as the risk of Fetal Varicella Syndrome is very low.

116 A 22- year- old Sudanese Asylum seeker is seen for booking in the antenatal clinic at 12 weeks. She is a primigravida and an ultrasound scan revealed a singleton pregnancy appropriate for gestation. She has history of female genital mutilation (FGM) and examination reveals Type II FGM.

What would be the he most appropriate management?

A. Defibulation during first stage of labour

B. Defibulation during second stage of labour

C. Elective caesarean section at 38 weeks to avoid labour

D. Elective defibulation at 20 weeks

E. Episiotomy only for second stage

GTG 53 Female Genital Mutilation and its Management

Defibulation can be carried out in the antenatal or intra-partum. Antenatal defibrillation should be carried out around 20 weeks and is preferred as it reduces risk of inexperienced care as an emergency in labour. A senior obstetrician with adequate experience should perform the defibulation.

117 A gravida 2 Para 1 + 0 attends the antenatal clinic for booking at 14 weeks. Her previous pregnancy was an emergency caesarean section for abruption at 38 weeks. Dating scan confirms a live fetus with a low risk for Down's syndrome. Routine bloods indicate her to have blood group B Rh negative and the antibody titre performed 2 weeks prior to the appointment reveals the anti-D level to be 5 IU/ml.

With regards to hemolytic disease of the fetus and newborn (HDFN), what is the optimal management?

A. Arrange for her partner's blood group to be tested for his Rhesus status

B. Enquire if she received anti-D following the previous pregnancy and delivery

C. Make a referral for fetal medicine opinion due to risk of HDFN

D. Reassure the mother that the HDFN is unlikely at that level and advice repeat assessment at 28 weeks

E. Repeat the blood test in 2 weeks to assess the anti-D levels again

GTG 65 The Management of Women with Red Cell Antibodies During Pregnancy

Anti-D levels of >4 IU/ml but <15 IU/ml correlates with a moderate risk of HDFN and therefore a referral for fetal medicine opinion should be made for levels >4 IU/ml. Once referral to metal medicine specialist has been made, for moderate risk of HDFN, the need for further quantification of anti-D levels is questionable. However, anti- D levels <4 IU/ml are considered to be of low risk for HDFN and immediate fetal medicine referral is not indicated. In such women, once detected, anti-D levels should be measured 4 weekly till 28 weeks and 2 weekly until delivery.

118 A primigravida complains of recurrent herpes at 32 weeks gestation. She has been treated with Aciclovir at 20 weeks for a primary episode of genital herpes. She would opt for caesarean section if Herpes lesions are detected at the onset of labour.

What would you advise?

A. Administer intravenous Aciclovir now and arrange elective caesarean at 39 weeks

B. Advise supportive treatment only for now and daily suppressive Acyclovir from 36 weeks

C. Advise supportive treatment only for now and intravenous therapy during labour

D. Reassure that the risk of neonatal herpes is very small and discharge back to midwife care

E. Repeat another course of oral Aciclovir and advice intravenous therapy during labour

GTG 30 Management of Genital Herpes in Pregnancy

Antiviral treatment is rarely advised for recurrent HSV as they are self-limiting and resolve within 7–10 days. Intravenous acyclovir is advised only for disseminated primary HSV antenatally or during labour for those who develop primary HSV within 6 weeks of EDD. While there is insufficient evidence to use daily suppressive acilocvir following one episode of primary HSV, it is recommended for those with a history of recurrent lesions during pregnancy to reduce the occurrence of HSV lesions at term – in particular if the mother would opt for caesarean in the presence of lesions during labour.

119 A primigravida is seen for booking. She is 40 years and has conceived through IVF. Ultrasound scan has confirmed a twin pregnancy. Her BMI is 36 kg/m^2.

What treatment would you advise to reduce the risk of pre-eclampsia?

A. Aspirin 75 mg daily
B. Folic acid 5 mg/day
C. Low molecular heparin 40 mg subcutaneously daily
D. Low salt diet
E. Vitamin C & E

NICE CG 107 Hypertension in Pregnancy

Women with one 'high risk' factor such as hypertensive disease during a previous pregnancy, chronic kidney disease, autoimmune disease such as systemic lupus erythematosus or antiphospholipid syndrome, Type 1 or Type 2 diabetes, or chronic hypertension should take Aspirin 75 mg daily from 12 weeks till delivery. Those with 2 or more moderate risk factors such as first pregnancy, age 40 years or older, pregnancy interval of more than 10 years, BMI of 35 kg/m^2 or more at first visit, family history of pre-eclampsia or multiple pregnancy should also be advised the same. Other medications are not effective and salt restriction should not be advised to prevent pre-eclampsia.

120 A community midwife requests advice with regard to induction of labour for a woman who is currently 40 weeks gestation. She has had 2 previous vaginal deliveries at 38 and 39 weeks. The pregnancy has been uncomplicated.

What would you advise?

A. To arrange induction as soon as possible
B. To arrange induction between 41–42 weeks and discuss membrane sweep

C. To arrange induction with amniotomy at 41 weeks

D. To continue expectant management even after 42 weeks with fetal surveillance until labour commences

E. To observe for 10 days and call again if the mother had not delivered

NICE CG 70 Induction of Labour

Women with uncomplicated pregnancies should usually be offered induction of labour between $41 + 0$ and $42 + 0$ weeks to avoid the risks of prolonged pregnancy. The exact timing should take into account the woman's preferences and local circumstances.

121 A gravida 2 Para 1, booked for low-risk midwifery care presents at 38 weeks with diminished fetal movements for 48 hours. The fetal heart rate was undetectable and sadly, intrauterine fetal death was confirmed with an ultrasound scan. The mother would prefer to go home and return 24 hours later for induction after arranging childcare for her other child. Her blood group is B RhD negative. What would you advise?

A. Advise 200 mg of mifepristone and then allow to go home

B. Advise a Kleihauer test and administer anti-RhD gamma globulin and allow to go home

C. Advise Kleihauer test to detect feto-maternal haemorrhage and allow to go home

D. Advise against going home

E. Allow her to go home

GTG 55 Late Intrauterine Fetal Death and Stillbirth

Major feto-maternal haemorrhage (FMH) is a silent cause of ntra uterine Fetal Death and a Kleihauer test is recommended for all women to diagnose the cause of fetal death. In RhD-negative women, the sensitising bleed that might have occurred days before death is diagnosed and in the above scenario at least 2 days prior to presentation. The window for optimal timing to prevent sensitisation is 72 hours as the benefit is reduced after that time period. Therefore, in such women anti-D gammaglobulin should be administered as soon as possible after presentation and Kleihauer test should be repeated at 48 hours to ensure that the fetal red cells have cleared, in particular if the FMH had been large – usually the case if the fetus dies in utero.

122 A British born primigravida with an uncomplicated pregnancy at 22 weeks gestation, needs to travel to sub-Saharan Africa for a family emergency and is expected to spend up to a month in Nigeria.

She wishes to know about the risk of contracting malaria.

What is her risk during a 1-month stay without chemo-prophylaxis?

A. 1:5000

B. 1:2500

C. 1:500

D. 1:50

E. 1:20

GTG 54a The Prevention of Malaria in Pregnancy

The risk of contracting malaria is dependent on the level of transmission and the season (dry vs rainy), rural or urban and the length of stay. The risk of contracting malaria during a one month stay without chemoprophylaxis in Sub-Saharan Africa is 1:50 – High.

123 A primigravida is seen in the antenatal clinic. A routine mid trimester anomaly scan at 20 weeks reveals an anterior placenta covering the os.

What is the most appropriate management?

A. Arrange a colour flow doppler scan

B. Arrange an MRI as soon as possible

C. Arrange a transvaginal scan immediately as it will reclassify unto 60% of the cases

D. Reassure the mother and arrange a repeat scan for placental localisation at 36 weeks

E. Reassure the mother that there is no need for any further investigations as the placenta will migrate upward as the pregnancy progresses

GTG 27 Placenta Previa, Placenta Accreta and Vasa Previa: Diagnosis and Management

Asymptomatic women with the placental edge leading up to the os can be managed expectantly with repeat imaging at 36 weeks gestation. Placenta covering the so at 20 weeks is considered to be a major degree and follow-up imaging is required. Large majority of routine mid trimester anomaly scans are transabdominal and ideally a transvaginal scan in the second trimester is indicated as this will reclassify up to 60% of the cases thus avoiding unnecessary follow-up. MRI and colour flow doppler can be useful but expensive.

124 A gravida 3 Para 2 is diagnosed with an anterior placenta reaching to the os at 20 weeks. She has had 2 previous caesarean sections. What further investigation would you arrange?
A. **Colour flow Doppler scan at 32 weeks**
B. MRI scan at 36 weeks
C. No further investigations
D. Transvaginal scan at 32 weeks
E. Ultrasound scan at 36 weeks for placental localisation

GTG 27 Placenta Previa, Placenta Accreta and Vasa Previa: Diagnosis and Management

Morbidly adherent placenta is a major risk if the mother had previous caesarean section. The risk is up to 40% in women who have had 2 previous caesareans. These women are also at a high risk of preterm delivery and the recommendation is to establish the diagnosis at 32 weeks with colour flow doppler. MRI is reserved only if the scan is equivocal.

125 A 29-year-old primigravida with a low-risk pregnancy attends the obstetric assessment unit with generalzsed pruritus at 34 weeks. What is the most important investigation to establish a diagnosis of obstetric cholestasis?
A. Bile acids and liver function tests
B. **Bile acids and liver function tests with pregnancy-specific reference ranges**
C. Coagulation status of the mother
D. Presenting symptoms of the mother
E. Ultrasound estimation of fetal weight

GTG 43 Obstetric Cholestasis

Obstetric cholestasis is diagnosed when otherwise unexplained pruritis occurs in pregnancy. Abnormal liver function tests with raised bile acid are considered sufficient for diagnosis. However, pregnancy-specific ranges for liver function tests should be used. Abnormalities in transaminases and gamma glutamyl transferase are significant. Increase in alkaline phosphatase is of placental origin and on its own does not indicate liver disease.

126 A multiparous woman is admitted to a delivery suite at 37 weeks gestation. She has been feeling unwell for the last 48 hours. She gives history of flu-like symptoms with cough, abdominal pain and watery vaginal discharge. Her temperature is 38, pulse 110 per minute, Respiratory rate 24 per minute. You have made a diagnosis of sepsis and antibiotics have been commenced after blood culture. Her serum lactate is 4 mmol/l.

What would be recommended for immediate intravenous fluid resuscitation?

A. Colloid 500 ml

B. Crystalloid 1000 ml

C. Crystalloid 20 ml/kg body weight

D. Crystalloid 40 ml/kg body weight

E. CVP line and fluid as required

GTG 64a Sepsis in Pregnancy

1. Obtain blood cultures prior to antibiotic administration
2. Administer broad-spectrum antibiotic within 1 hour of recognition of severe sepsis
3. Measure serum lactate
4. In the event of hypotension and/or a serum lactate >4 mmol/l, deliver an initial minimum 20 ml/kg of crystalloid or an equivalent
5. Apply vasopressors for hypotension that is not responding to initial fluid resuscitation to maintain mean arterial pressure (MAP) > 65 mmHg
6. In the event of persistent hypotension despite fluid resuscitation (septic shock) and/or lactate > 4 mmol/l
   a. Achieve a central venous pressure (CVP) of ≥8 mmHg
   b. Achieve central venous oxygen saturation (ScvO2) ≥ 70% or mixed venous oxygen saturation (ScvO2) ≥ 65%.

127 A primigravida aged 37 is seen at booking. This is a pregnancy following assisted conception. Her BMI is 19 and the ultrasound scan has confirmed a singleton fetus appropriate for the period of gestation.

What is the recommended investigation to identify fetus at risk of SGA age?

A. 2-weekly liquor volume and uterine artery Doppler from 26 weeks

B. 3-weekly serial ultrasound scan for growth and estimated fetal weight from 28 week onwards

C. Detailed anomaly scan to be performed by a fetal medicine specialist at 20 weeks to look for fetal echogenic bowel

D. Growth scans at 28 and 34 weeks

E. Uterine artery Doppler at 20–24 weeks

GTG 31 The Investigation and Management of Small for Gestational Age Fetus

It is recommended that all women should be assessed at booking for risk factors for an SGA fetus to identify the need for increased surveillance. In high-risk populations, uterine artery Doppler at 20–24 weeks of pregnancy has a moderate predictive value for a severely SGA neonate. Women who have one major risk factor or three or more minor risk factors (as in the given scenario) should be referred for uterine artery Doppler at 20–24 weeks of gestation. The risk of SGA is high even if the uterine artery Doppler normalises later on in pregnancy. Therefore, women with abnormal uterine artery Doppler at 20–14 weeks should have serial ultrasound for growth and Doppler from 26 weeks at 2–3 weekly interval.

128 A 40-year-old primigravida is seen in the antenatal clinic with a twin pregnancy conceived through IVF. Gestation is 11 + 6 days and the ultrasound scan has confirmed DCDA twins appropriate for the gestation with normal nuchal thickening.

What is the appropriate monitoring to detect growth discordance?

A. Growth scans at 28 and 34 weeks

B. Serial growth scans every 2 weeks from 20 weeks

C. Serial growth scans with fetal weight estimation every 2 weeks from 16 weeks

D. Serial growth scans with fetal weight estimation every 3–4 weeks from 20 weeks

E. Symphysio-fundal measurement

NICE CG 129 Multiple Pregnancy

Fetal weight discordance using two or more biometric parameters at each ultrasound scan from 20 weeks is recommended at intervals of less than 28 days. A 25% or greater difference in size between twins or triplets as a clinically important indicator of intrauterine growth restriction and referral to a tertiary level fetal medicine centre is indicated. Two weekly scans from sixteen weeks are recommended for monochorionic twins.

129 A 38-year-old gravida 3 Para 2 is admitted at 32 week gestation feeling unwell. She has been gradually becoming more anxious through the day with cough and chest pain, which was worse during inspiration. Observations are as follows:

Temperature 37.2 °C, Pulse 110 per minute, BP 98/60, RR 24 per minute and blood gases reveal mild respiratory alkalosis.

What is the most appropriate management plan?

A. Perform an urgent chest X-ray and electrocardiogram and commence the patient on therapeutic unfractionated heparin infusion

B. Perform an urgent chest X-ray and electrocardiogram and commence the patient on therapeutic low molecular weight heparin

C. Request a ventilation-perfusion scan to rule out pulmonary embolism

D. Request an urgent computed tomography pulmonary angiogram to rule out pulmonary embolism

E. Take blood cultures and start the patient on intravenous antibiotics

GTG 37b The Acute Management of Thrombosis and Embolism During Pregnancy and Puerperium.

Any pregnant woman with symptoms and/or signs suggestive of venous thromboembolism should have objective testing performed urgently and treatment with low molecular weight heparin should be commenced until the diagnosis is excluded by objective testing.

130 A 37-year-old primigravida weighing 102 kg (BMI 40 kg/m²) is seen in an antenatal clinic for booking. She conceived via assisted conception following a long period of subfertility. Ultrasound has confirmed a dichorionic diamniotic twin pregnancy of 11 + 5 days gestation.

What is the best practice with regard to reducing maternal risk of venous thromboembolism?

A. Advise compression stockings and mobilisation throughout pregnancy

B. Commence 75 mg of Aspirin per day and advice good hydration and mobilisation

C. Consider and advise low molecular weight heparin – Enoxaparin 40 mg per day throughout pregnancy

D. Consider and advise low molecular weight heparin – Enoxaparin 60 mg per day throughout pregnancy

E. Consider and advise unfractionated heparin daily throughout pregnancy

GTG 37a Reducing Risk of Thrombosis and Embolism During Pregnancy and Puerperium.

Any woman with four or more antenatal risk factors (age > 35, BMI > 30 kg/m^2, assisted conception and multiple pregnancy as above) should be considered for prophylactic mow molecular weight heparin throughout the antenatal period and for 6 weeks in the postnatal period after a postnatal risk assessment. The dose recommendation for maternal weight of 91–130 kg is 60 mg Enoxaparin/day. Alternatively, 9000 units of Tinzaparin/day or 10,000 units of Daltaparin/day can be prescribed.

Module 9

Maternal Medicine

131 A woman with chronic essential hypertension was converted from Lisinopril to methyldopa in a preconception counselling clinic.
The pregnancy was uncomplicated and she delivered spontaneously at term.
At what stage postnatally should the antihypertensive medication be switched back to Lisinopril?

A. 2 days
B. 7 days
C. 14 days
D. 6 weeks
E. 12 weeks

NICE CG 107 Hypertension in Pregnancy

If a woman has taken methyldopa to treat chronic hypertension during pregnancy, stop within 2 days of birth and restart the antihypertensive treatment the woman was taking before she planned the pregnancy.

132 A 32-year-old woman primigravida who is 34 weeks pregnant attends the antenatal clinic complaining of severe itching.
Serum bile acids are found to be elevated and she is diagnosed with obstetric cholestasis.
What is the most effective medication to improve her itching?

A. Activated charcoal
B. Chlorphenamine
C. Colestyramine
D. S-adenosyl methionine
E. Ursodeoxycholic acid

Part 2 MRCOG: Single Best Answer Questions, First Edition.
Andrew Sizer, Chandrika Balachandar, Nibedan Biswas, Richard Foon, Anthony Griffiths, Sheena Hodgett, Banchhita Sahu and Martyn Underwood.
© 2016 John Wiley & Sons, Ltd. Published 2016 by John Wiley & Sons, Ltd.

GTG 43 Obstetric Cholestasis

Systemic treatments aimed at relieving pruritus include colestyramine, a poorly tolerated bile acid-chelating agent, which may improve pruritus in some women but may also exacerbate vitamin K deficiency (which has been associated with fetal intracranial haemorrhage). Colestyramine has not been subjected to randomised trials and is not in clinical use. Antihistamines such as chlorphenamine may provide some welcome sedation at night but do not have a significant impact on pruritus. Activated charcoal and guar gum do not relieve pruritus.

There is insufficient evidence to demonstrate whether S-adenosylmethionine (SAMe) is effective for either control of maternal symptoms or for improving fetal outcome, and it is therefore not recommended.

Ursodeoxycholic acid (UDCA) improves pruritus and liver function in women with obstetric cholestasis.

133 What is the main contraindication to the use of antenatal corticosteroids?
A. Chorioamnionitis
B. Cushing's syndrome
C. Diabetes mellitus
D. Multiple pregnancy
E. Systemic infection

GTG 7 Antenatal Corticosteroids to Reduce Neonatal Morbidity and Mortality

Caution should be exercised when giving corticosteroid therapy to women with systemic infection including tuberculosis or sepsis.

In cases of chorioamnionitis, a course of antenatal corticosteroids may be administered, but should not delay delivery if indicated by maternal or fetal condition.

Diabetes mellitus is not a contraindication to antenatal corticosteroid treatment for fetal lung maturation.

134 In the recent MBRRACE-UK report (2014), what was the leading overall single cause of maternal death?
A. Cardiac disease
B. Haemorrhage
C. Sepsis
D. Suicide
E. Thromboembolism

Saving Lives, Improving Mothers' Care
Lessons learned to inform future maternity care from the United
Kingdom and Ireland Confidential Enquiries into Maternal Deaths and
Morbidity 2009–2012.

As in previous reports, cardiac disease remains the largest single cause
of indirect maternal deaths.

135 An anaesthetist is asked to assist with the insertion of an intravenous cannula prior to the commencement of a Syntocinon infusion in labour.

The cannula is inserted successfully, but shortly after it was flushed
through as the woman starts to have convulsions and becomes
hypotensive and bradycardic.

The syringes on the trolley are unlabeled and the anaesthetist suspects he may have flushed the cannula with a local anaesthetic
solution.

What is the appropriate management of her collapse?
A. Activated charcoal orally
B. Calcium gluconate 10% IV
C. Intralipid 20% infusion
D. Magnesium sulphate 20% IV
E. Potassium chloride 10% IV

**GTG 56 Maternal Collapse in Pregnancy
and the Puerperium**
If local anaesthetic toxicity is suspected, stop injecting immediately.

Lipid rescue should be used in cases of collapse secondary to local
anaesthetic toxicity.

Intralipid 20% should be available in all maternity units.

136 A 32-year-old woman with known HIV-1 infection is being
seen in antenatal clinic in her first pregnancy. Her viral load
is <50 copies/ml at 36 weeks gestation and she wishes to have
further pregnancies in the future.

What is the most significant intervention to reduce mother to child
transmission?
A. Avoiding invasive procedures during delivery
B. Elective caesarean section at term
C. Exclusive replacement feeding of the baby
D. Initiation of antiretroviral therapy during pregnancy
E. Mixed feeding of the baby

TOG Article
Byrne L, Fakoya A, Harding K. HIV in pregnancy. TOG 2012;14:17–24.
HAART is the single most important intervention in reducing mother to child transmission.

137 Prior to the development of highly active antiretroviral therapy (HAART), elective caesarean section was the standard mode of delivery to reduce intrapartum mother to child transmission of HIV.

At what viral load should caesarean section be considered with present HAART management?

A. 0–50 copies/ml

B. 50–400 copies/ml

C. 400–500 copies/ml

D. 500–600 copies/ml

E. 600–700 copies/ml

TOG Article
Byrne L, Fakoya A, Harding K. HIV in pregnancy. TOG 2012;14:17–24.
If the maternal viral load is undetectable at 36 weeks, a vaginal delivery can be planned. Women on zidovudine monotherapy and those on HAART (or START) with a detectable viral load at 36 weeks (>400 copies/ml) are recommended to have elective caesarean section at 38 weeks. A caesarean section should be considered in those with a viral load 50–400 copies/ml.

138 With the present multidisciplinary management of HIV in pregnancy using HAART, what is the rate of mother to child transmission of HIV in the United Kingdom?

A. 0.3%

B. 0.7%

C. 1.5%

D. 3%

E. 6%

TOG Article
Byrne L, Fakoya A, Harding K. HIV in pregnancy. TOG 2012;14:17–24.
In the United Kingdom, the rate of mother to child transmission of HIV in women on HAART is 0.7% with both elective caesarean section and vaginal delivery.

M9 MATERNAL MEDICINE

139 A woman who is HIV positive attends antenatal clinic at 36 weeks gestation. She has an uncomplicated pregnancy.

At what plasma viral load could vaginal delivery be recommended?

A. Less than 50 HIV RNA copies/ml

B. Less than 100 HIV RNA copies/ml

C. Less than 150 HIV RNA copies/ml

D. Less than 200 HIV RNA copies/ml

E. Less than 250 HIV RNA copies/ml

British HIV Association Guidelines for the Management of HIV Infection in Pregnant Women (2014 Interim Review)

For women taking combined ART, a decision regarding the recommended mode of delivery should be made after a review of plasma viral load results at 36 weeks.

For women with a plasma viral load of <50 HIV RNA copies/ml at 36 weeks, and in the absence of obstetric contraindications, a planned vaginal delivery is recommended.

For women with a plasma viral load of 50–399 HIV RNA copies/ml at 36 weeks, PLCS (Planned elective caesarean section) should be considered, taking into account the actual viral load, the trajectory of the viral load, length of time on treatment, adherence issues, obstetric factors and the woman's views.

Where the viral load is ≥400 HIV RNA copies/ml at 36 weeks, PLCS is recommended.

In women for whom a vaginal delivery has been recommended and labour has commenced, obstetric management should follow the same guidelines as for the uninfected population.

140 A 29-year-old primigravida attends her booking visit at 12 + 2 days. An ultrasound scan has confirmed a live fetus appropriate for the period of gestation. She is known to be HIV positive and is not in need of treatment for her own health, with a viral load of >35,000 copies/ml and is very keen for a vaginal delivery.

What is the most appropriate intervention with regards to reducing the risk of neonatal transmission of HIV?

A. Advise against vaginal delivery and recommend elective LSCS at 38 weeks

B. Initiate cART at the beginning of second trimester weeks and to be discontinued at delivery

C. Initiate cART immediately and continued for 6 weeks postpartum

D. Initiate Zidovudine monotherapy immediately and continue for 6 weeks postpartum

E. Initiate Zidovudine monotherapy immediately and discontinue at delivery

British HIV Association Guidelines for the Management of HIV Infection in Pregnant Women 2012 (2014 Interim Review)

Women who do not require treatment for themselves should commence temporary cART at the beginning of the second trimester if the baseline viral load is >30,000 copies/ml and earlier if viral load is >100,000 copies/ml. Zidovudine monotherapy is only advised for those opting for elective LSCS and have a baseline viral load of <10,000 copies/ml.

141 A 29-year-old gravida 2 para 1 is admitted with history of preterm prelabour rupture of membranes at 31 + 5 weeks gestation of 4 hours duration. She is a known HIV patient with a low viral load and had been commenced on HAART at 22 weeks. Her viral load at 28 weeks was <50 copies/ml. On admission, she is apyrexial, vital signs are within normal limits and the CTG is reassuring.

What is the most appropriate immediate management with regard to delivery?

A. **Undertake genital infection screen, rapid testing for current viral load, administer steroids and oral erythromycin and arrange MDT consultation**

B. Undertake genital infection screen, rapid testing of current viral load, commence broad-spectrum antibiotics and arrange for category 1 LSCS

C. Undertake genital infection screen, rapid testing of current viral load, commence broad-spectrum antibiotic and arrange for category 2 LSCS

D. Undertake genital infection screen, rapid testing of current viral load, commence broad-spectrum antibiotics and arrange for category 3 LSCS

E. Undertake genital infection screen and rapid testing for current viral load, administer steroids and induce labour after 48 hours

British HIV Association Guidelines for the Management of HIV Infection in Pregnant Women 2012 (2014 Interim Review)

When PPROM occurs before 34 weeks in patients receiving cART and there is no evidence of chorio-amnionitis and/or metal distress, the decision to expedite delivery should be made after MDT consultation. In such patients, oral erythromycin and steroid administration should be as for the general population.

142 A 29-year-old gravida 2 para 1 is seen in an antenatal clinic at 37 weeks for the first time. She has transferred her booking from another region, where she had been diagnosed as HIV positive. Her viral load is 1000 copies/ml. She does not need treatment for her own health and was started on zidovudine monotherapy at the previous hospital. Her previous delivery was spontaneous vaginal delivery with no complications.

What is the most appropriate management plan for delivery?

A. Advise to continue zidovudine therapy and arrange elective caesarean at 38 weeks with intravenous zidovudine cover for delivery to be discontinued at delivery

B. Advise to continue zidovudine therapy and arrange elective caesarean at 38 weeks with intravenous cover for delivery and change over to cART after delivery

C. Advise to continue zidovudine therapy and await spontaneous labour with intravenous zidovudine cover during labour and discontinue at delivery

D. Stop zidovudine and initiate cART and arrange for elective caesarean section at 38 weeks and discontinue treatment at delivery

E. Stop zidovudine and initiate cART and await spontaneous labour and discontinue treatment at delivery

British HIV Association Guidelines for the Management of HIV Infection in Pregnant Women 2012 (2014 Interim Review)

Option of Zidovudine monotherapy for those with viral load of less than 10,000 copies/ml can only be given along with the option of elective LSCS between 38 and 39 weeks. It is administered orally and intravenous cover for delivery is recommended. Zidovudine is less toxic than cART and has been shown to significantly reduce mother to child transmission with LSCS as the mode of delivery. If the mother does not need treatment for her own health, medication can be stopped at delivery.

143 A young primigravida attends assessment unit at 32 weeks gestation following an assessment of raised blood pressure by the community midwife. Urine protein: creatinine ratio is 32 mg/mmol and her blood pressure is 152/102 mmHg.

What is the most appropriate management plan?

A. **Admit and commence antihypertensive treatment**

B. Admit for observation with 6-hourly blood pressure monitoring and daily protein: creatinine ratio

C. Admit for observation

D. Discharge back to community midwife with advice for blood pressure and automated reagent-strip test for proteinuria twice weekly

E. Discharge back to community midwife with advice for blood pressure and urine protein: creatinine ratio on a daily basis

NICE CG 107 Hypertension in Pregnancy

Blood pressure of 150/100–159/109 is considered moderate hypertension and spot urine protein: creatinine ratio of >30 mg/mmol is pre-eclampsia. Such patients should be admitted and antihypertensive treatment with labetalol as first line therapy should be commenced to maintain the systolic blood pressure below 150 mm of Hg and diastolic between 80 and 100 mm/Hg.

144 A primigravida with a BMI of 34 kg/m^2 presents at 21 weeks gestation with severe throbbing headache and vomiting. She gives a history of similar headaches in the past. On examination, her blood pressure is found to be normal with no proteinuria and the deep tendon reflexes are normal. A neurological review is arranged as there are no localising neurological signs except mild bilateral sixth nerve paresis.

What is the most likely diagnosis?

A. **Benign idiopathic intracranial hypertension**

B. Depression

C. Migraine

D. Pre-eclampsia

E. Space occupying lesion

TOG Article

Thirumalaikumar L, Ramalingam K, Heafield T. Idiopathic intracranial hypertension in pregnancy. The Obstetrician & Gynaecologist 2014;16:93–97.

Idiopathic intracranial hypertension has a female to male ratio of 8:1. The incidence in women of child-bearing age is 0.9/100,000 but increases to 19.3/100,000 in obese women. Presentation is usually severe throbbing retro-bulbar headache usually in the first half of the pregnancy but can present in the third trimester. Fundoscopy will reveal papilloedema and neuro-imaging is essential to exclude other causes. Benign idiopathic intracranial hypertension is a diagnosis of exclusion.

145 A primigravida has been brought to the Accident and Emergency department following a road traffic accident at 32 weeks gestation. The obstetric registrar is summoned urgently. On arrival she learns that CPR had been commenced 3 minutes earlier following a diagnosis of cardiac arrest and pulseless electrical activity.
What is the most appropriate initial action for an ST5 trainee?
A. Advise ALS algorithm
B. Advise Dexamethasone for fetal lung maturity
C. Arrange transfer to delivery suite for category 1 caesarean section
D. Call the consultant
E. Prepare and commence caesarean section with the aim to achieve delivery within 5 minutes of maternal collapse

GTG 56 Maternal Collapse in Pregnancy and Puerperium

If there is no response to correctly performed CPR within 4 minutes of maternal collapse in women beyond 20 weeks gestation, delivery should be achieved within 5 minutes to assist maternal resuscitation. The rationale for this is that the pregnant woman becomes hypoxic faster than nonpregnant women and irreversible brain damage can occur within 4–6 minutes. Delivery of the fetus and placenta improves cardiac output by increasing the venous return and reduces oxygen consumption. It also facilitates chest compression and makes ventilation easier. Though delivery within 5 minutes improves survival chances for the baby, in the interest of the mother this has to be undertaken even if the fetus is dead. Perimortem caesarean section should not be delayed by moving the mother. It should be performed where the resuscitation is taking place.

146 A primigravida aged 30 attends antenatal clinic at 34 weeks gestation. She is known to have mild bipolar disorder but has not required any medication prior to pregnancy. Her mother suffers from bipolar disorder and takes lithium. During the visit she reports increasing anxiety, depression and self-neglect.
To which health professional should this patient be referred?

A. Community midwife

B. Consultant Obstetrician

C. General Practitioner for appropriate medications

D. General Practitioner with advice for CPN Support

E. **Specialised perinatal mental health services or general psychiatry services as available**

RCOG – Good Practice 14 Management of Women with Mental Health Issues during Pregnancy and Postnatal period

Women at high risk of postpartum psychosis should be referred to specialised perinatal mental health services or general psychiatry services as available. Such women are those

- with current severe psychiatric symptoms
- with past history of serious postpartum illness or bipolar disorder or schizophrenia who develop moderate symptoms in pregnancy
- on complex psychotropic medications.

147 A 39-year-old Type 2 diabetic of Asian origin presents with an acute onset of epigastric pain, chest pain and breathlessness at 30 weeks gestation. She is gravida 5 Para 4 (four normal vaginal deliveries), and has a BMI of 41 kg/m². This was an unplanned pregnancy. Her diabetes is poorly controlled and her haemoglobin was 85 g/l at 28 weeks. She is on oral iron and there is history of familial hyperlipidemia.

What is the most likely working diagnosis for this mother?

A. **Acute myocardial infarction (AMI)**

B. Chest infection

C. Pulmonary embolism

D. Pulmonary edema

E. Rib flaring/musculoskeletal pain

TOG Article

Wuntakal R, Shetty N, Ioannou E, Sharma S, Kurian J. Myocardial infarction and pregnancy. The Obstetrician & Gynaecologist 2013; 15:247–255.

The symptoms described above in the presence of known AMI risk factors should be investigated further and a high index of suspicion is important as two consecutive CMACE reports have shown a consistent failure to consider AMI as a cause of chest pain in women with risk factors.

148 A 32-year-old primigravida is admitted in spontaneous early labour at 39 + 2 weeks. She is a known asthmatic and has had repeated admissions in this pregnancy with acute exacerbations of asthma. The previous admission had been at 36 weeks gestation when she was commenced on oral prednisolone 7.5 mg/day in view of persistent poor asthmatic control.

What is the most appropriate intervention to maintain asthma control in labour?

A. 100 mg of parenteral hydrocortisone 6–8 hourly during labour

B. Continuous oxygen by face mask

C. Deliver by caesarean section

D. Refer to a respiratory physician

E. Regular inhaled long-acting Beta 2 agonist along with her current medications

TOG Article

Goldie MH, Brightling CE. Asthma in pregnancy. The Obstetrician & Gynaecologist 2013;15:241–245.

Asthma control in pregnancy is variable and about 35% of pregnant asthmatics would experience worsening of the condition and 11–18% would have at least one visit to A&E and of these 62% might require admission. Mothers should be encouraged to continue their medication as poor control could result in poor obstetric outcome. Systemic steroids are recommended for maintaining control during labour.

149 A 29-year-old primigravida with a low-risk pregnancy attends the obstetric assessment unit with generalised pruritus at 34 weeks gestation. Laboratory results reveal bile acids of 16 mmol/l with normal Liver Function Tests (LFT) and you have established a diagnosis of Obstetric Cholestasis.

What is considered to be the best practice with regard to further antenatal care?

A. Reassure and continue with midwifery care along with weekly Bile acid and LFT estimation

B. Reassure and continue with midwifery care and arrange induction of labour at 37–38 weeks

C. Reassure and transfer booking to consultant-led care

D. Review mother in the assessment unit, discuss increased risk of stillbirth and arrange induction of labour at 37–38 weeks

E. Transfer booking to consultant-led care and arrange a clinic review with repeat bile acid and LFT estimation

GTG 43 Obstetric Cholestasis

Obstetric cholestasis is associated with an increased incidence of passage of meconium, premature delivery, fetal distress, delivery by caesarean section and postpartum haemorrhage. It is also associated with premature delivery – iatrogenic or otherwise. Therefore, it is recommended that women diagnosed with cholestasis should be booked and deliver in a consultant-led unit.

150 An 18-year-old primigravida is seen in the antenatal clinic for booking at 8 weeks gestation. She is known to have sickle cell disease and her partner is known to have normal haemoglobin. She has recently arrived from Nigeria and has not taken any vitamin supplements so far.

What is the most important vitamin supplement during pregnancy?

A. Folic acid 1 mg immediately for throughout pregnancy

B. Folic acid 400 µg immediately for throughout pregnancy

C. Folic acid 400 µg immediately until 12 weeks gestation

D. Folic acid 5 mg immediately for throughout pregnancy

E. Folic acid 5 mg immediately until 12 weeks gestation

GTG 61 Management of Sickle Cell Disease in Pregnancy

Sickle cell disease is a hemolytic anaemia and these women are at risk of folate deficiency. Folic acid of 1 mg is advised outside of pregnancy while 5 mg is recommended throughout pregnancy.

151 An 18-year-old primigravida, a recent immigrant from West Africa is admitted at 30 weeks gestation with severe pain in her hips. A diagnosis of acute painful sickle cell crisis has been made.

What is the most important immediate management?

A. Admission and rapid assessment followed by morphine for pain relief

B. Admission and rapid assessment followed by non-steroidal anti-inflammatory drugs

C. Admission and rapid assessment followed by oxygen and hydration without any analgesics

D. Admission and rapid assessment followed by Pethidine for pain relief

E. Observation and discharge home with Codeine and paracetamol

GTG 61 Management of Sickle Cell Disease in Pregnancy

Painful crisis is the most frequent complication of SCD with 27–50% of women experiencing a painful crisis in pregnancy. Strong opioid such as morphine is advised. Pethidine should be avoided due to associated risk of seizures. While fluid and oxygen might be needed, opioid analgesia is the most important immediate management.

152 A 31-year-old primigravida presents for booking at 10 weeks. She is known to be hypothyroid and is on Levothyroxine 75 μg. She is complaining of feeling tired and lethargic and her TSH is 6.5 mU/ml.

What would be the target TSH level at this gestation to indicate optimal control?

A. 0.1–2.5 mU/ml

B. 0.5–3.5 mU/m

C. 4.5 mU/ml is satisfactory

D. Just below 4.5 mU/ml

E. Obtain advice from an Endocrine Specialist

TOG Article

Jefferys A, Vanderpump M, Yasmin E. Thyroid dysfunction and reproductive health. The Obstetrician & Gynaecologist 2015;17:39–45.

Hypothyroidism is common with overt disease affecting 0.5% of women and subclinical disease affecting about 2.5%. Both are associated with adverse outcomes and adequate Levothyroxine replacement is essential to reduce these. Trimester-specific Thyroid Stimulating Hormone (TSH) range should be used to monitor adequacy of Levothyroxine replacement. Recommended TSH reference ranges are as follows:

First trimester	0.1–2.5 mU/ml
Second trimester	0.2–3.0 mU/ml
Third trimester	0.3–3.0 mU/ml

In women who are administered Levothyroxine before pregnancy, the dose should be increased initially by 25 μg daily once the pregnancy is confirmed and thyroid function tests should be repeated 4–6 weekly to maintain TSH levels within the above given reference ranges.

153 A 38-year-old pregnant woman with obesity and Type 2 diabetes presents with chest pain at 28 weeks gestation. Which is the blood marker of choice for diagnosis of AMI in pregnancy?

A. Creatine kinase isoenzyme MB
B. C-reactive protein
C. Lactate dehydrogenase
D. Myoglobin
E. Troponin

TOG Article

Wuntakal R, Shetty N, Ioannou E, Sharma S, Kurian J. Myocardial infarction in pregnancy. The Obstetrician & Gynaecologist 2013; 15:247–255.

Troponin is never increased in healthy pregnant women and is not affected by anaesthesia, prolonged labour or caesarean section unlike other cardiac markers, which may be significantly increased in labour.

154 Following diagnosis of AMI in pregnancy, which medication should not be used in the acute phase?
A. Aspirin
B. Labetalol
C. Low molecular weight heparin
D. Nifedipine
E. Unfractionated heparin

TOG Article

Wuntakal R, Shetty N, Ioannou E, Sharma S, Kurian J. Myocardial infarction in pregnancy. The Obstetrician & Gynaecologist 2013;15:247–255.

Nifedipine can be safely used in pregnancy; however, nifedipine should be avoided after an acute coronary event as it has been shown to increase mortality.

155 What is the approximate incidence of overt hypothyroidism in pregnancy?
A. 0.1%
B. 0.5%
C. 1.0%
D. 2.0%
E. 2.5%

TOG Article

Jefferys A, Vanderpump M, Yasmin E. Thyroid dysfunction and reproductive health. The Obstetrician & Gynaecologist 2015;17:39–45.

Hypothyroidism in pregnancy is a relatively common condition with overt disease affecting approximately 0.5% of women and subclinical disease approximately 2.5%.

156 A 41-year-old woman has an oral glucose tolerance test (OGTT) at 28 weeks gestation in her fourth pregnancy. The results are as follows:

Fasting plasma glucose: 5.8 mmol/l

2 hour plasma glucose: 7.4 mmol/l

What is the correct diagnosis?

A. Impaired glucose tolerance

B. Gestational diabetes

C. Maturity onset diabetes of the young (MODY)

D. Normal glycemic control

E. Type 2 diabetes

NICE 3 Diabetes in Pregnancy: Management of Diabetes and its Complications from Preconception to the Post Natal Period

Diagnose gestational diabetes if the woman has either:

- a fasting plasma glucose level of 5.6 mmol/l or above or
- a 2 hour plasma glucose level of 7.8 mmol/l or above.

157 A 30-year-old woman is diagnosed with gestational diabetes following an oral glucose tolerance test (OGGT) at 26 weeks gestation in her first pregnancy. Her fasting blood glucose is 7.2 mmol/l. What is the appropriate management?

A. Dietary modification alone

B. Dietary modification and exercise

C. Glibenclamide

D. Insulin

E. Metformin

NICE 3 Diabetes in Pregnancy: Management of Diabetes and its Complications from Preconception to the Post Natal Period

Offer immediate treatment with insulin, with or without metformin, as well as changes in diet and exercise, to women with gestational diabetes who have a fasting plasma glucose level of 7.0 mmol/l or above at diagnosis.

158 A 20-year-old woman with Type 1 diabetes presents at 32 weeks gestation in her first pregnancy with regular painful contractions, a closed cervix and a positive fetal fibronectin test. What is the most appropriate management plan?

A. Antenatal steroids

B. Antenatal steroids and additional insulin

C. Antenatal steroids and tocolysis with atosiban

D. Antenatal steroids, additional insulin and tocolysis with atosiban

E. Tocolysis with atosiban

NICE 3 Diabetes in Pregnancy: Management of Diabetes and Its Complications from Preconception to the Post Natal Period

In preterm labour, diabetes should not be considered a contraindication to antenatal steroids for fetal lung maturation or to tocolysis.

In women with insulin-treated diabetes who are receiving steroids for fetal lung maturation, give additional insulin according to an agreed protocol and monitor them closely.

159 What is the prevalence of asthma in pregnant women?

A. 0.1–0.4%

B. 0.5–1%

C. 2–3%

D. 4–12%

E. 14–20%

TOG Article

Goldie M, Brightling C. Asthma in pregnancy. The Obstetrician & Gynaecologist 2013;15:241–245.

The prevalence of asthma in pregnant women is 4–12% making it the most common chronic condition in pregnancy.

160 For women with severe asthma, in what proportion does disease further deteriorate during pregnancy?

A. 10%

B. 30%

C. 40%

D. 50%

E. 60%

TOG Article
Goldie M, Brightling C. Asthma in pregnancy. The Obstetrician & Gynaecologist 2013;15:241–245.

In severe disease, asthma control is more likely to deteriorate (~60%) than in mild disease (~10%).

161 For which group of women is vitamin K supplementation advised in the last month of pregnancy?
    A. Women taking anti-epileptic drugs
    B. Women with two or more risk factors for pre-eclampsia
    C. Women with a body mass index (BMI) > 35
    D. Women with liver disease
    E. Women with pre-existing diabetes

TOG Article
Duckworth S, Mistry H, Chappell L. Vitamin supplementation in pregnancy. The Obstetrician & Gynaecologist 2012;14:175–178.

National guidelines (Scottish Intercollegiate Guidelines Network) recommend that oral vitamin K should be given in the last month of pregnancy, only in those with risk factors for haemorrhagic disease of the newborn (maternal liver disease, anticipated premature delivery).

162 A woman with a BMI of 40 whose epilepsy is well controlled on anti-epileptic drugs (AEDs) attends for a booking appointment with the community midwife at 10 weeks gestation. Which combination of vitamin supplements should she be advised to take?
    A. Folic acid 400 mcg and vitamin D 10 mcg
    B. Folic acid 400 mcg and vitamin K 10 mg
    C. Folic acid 5 mg and vitamin C 70 mg
    D. Folic acid 5 mg and vitamin D 10 mcg
    E. Vitamin D 10 mcg and vitamin C 70 mg

TOG Article
Duckworth S, Mistry H, Chappell L. Vitamin supplementation in pregnancy. The Obstetrician & Gynaecologist 2012;14:175–178.

Current NICE guidelines endorse the use of 5 mg/day of folic acid supplementation from pre-pregnancy in women taking AEDs.

NICE acknowledges the importance of improved maternal awareness of vitamin D supplementation of 10 mcg/day in the following high-risk women who have a pre-pregnancy BMI of >30.

163 A woman who is taking antipsychotic medication is contemplating pregnancy.

Why is Lithium not the drug of choice?

A. Risk of cardiac defects in the fetus

B. Risk of constipation in the fetus

C. Risk of gestational diabetes

D. Risk of maternal hypertension

E. Possible risk of neonatal persistent pulmonary hypertension

SIGN Guideline 60 Postnatal depression and puerperal psychosis

Lithium in pregnancy increases the risk of

- Fetal heart defects
- Ebstein's anomaly
- Neurological effects including CNS and respiratory complications if exposed to high levels during delivery.
- Neonatal toxicity; floppy baby syndrome and hypothyroidism.

164 A woman is recently diagnosed with gestational diabetes. A programme of exercise and dietary change is initiated. What is the likelihood of her needing further treatment with an oral hypoglycemic agent or insulin therapy in this pregnancy?

A. 1–2%

B. 10–20%

C. 30–40%

D. 80%+

E. 90%+

NICE CG 62 Antenatal Care

In most women, gestational diabetes will respond to changes in diet and exercise.

Some women (between 10% and 20%) will need oral hypoglycemic agents or insulin therapy if diet and exercise are not effective in controlling gestational diabetes.

165 A woman attends the perimental health antenatal clinic at 8 weeks of gestation. She wishes to stop her lithium therapy with the support of her psychiatrist and seeks advice.

What should be the recommended action after fully counselling the patient?

A. Immediately stop lithium therapy due to its high teratogenic risks

B. Mandatory to continue in pregnancy due to the high risk of mania

C. Stop gradually over the next 4 weeks to reduce the risk of mania

D. Stop immediately but convert to Carbamazepine

E. Stop only if patient agrees to accept an additional antipsychotic treatment

NICE CG 192 Antenatal and Postnatal Mental Health

If a woman taking lithium becomes pregnant, consider stopping the drug gradually over 4 weeks if she is well. Explain to her that

- stopping medication may not remove the risk of fetal heart malformations
- there is a risk of relapse, particularly in the postnatal period, if she has bipolar disorder.

166 A woman attends clinic for preconceptual counselling after previously being treated for breast carcinoma. She is planning a pregnancy. How long after completion of the treatment is it recommended to wait before conceiving?

A. 1 month

B. 6 months

C. 1 year

D. 2 years

E. 3 years

GTG 12 Pregnancy and Breast Cancer

Women are generally advised to wait for at least 2 years after treatment for breast cancer before conception because of the risk of early relapse. The rate of disease recurrence is highest in the first 3 years after diagnosis and then declines, although late relapses do occur up to 10 years and more from the time of diagnosis.

167 A primagravida who is otherwise fit and well, sadly, has a stillbirth at 38 weeks of gestation.

In what proportion of cases is there no identifiable cause?

A. Almost 10% of cases

B. Almost 30% of cases

C. Almost 50% of cases

D. Almost 70% of cases

E. Almost 90% of cases

GTG 55 Late Intrauterine Fetal Death and Stillbirth

Parents should be advised that no specific cause is found in almost half of stillbirths.

168 A woman with known sickle cell trait attends an antenatal booking clinic.

What antenatal complication is significantly more common compared to uncomplicated pregnancies?

A. Chest infection

B. Intrauterine growth restriction

C. Major postpartum haemorrhage

D. Placental abruption

E. Urinary tract infection

TOG Article

Eissa AA, Tuck SM. Sickle cell disease and β-thalassaemia major in pregnancy. The Obstetrician & Gynaecologist 2013;15:71–78.

Pregnancy in women with sickle cell trait has few additional complication rates compared with other women of the same ethnic and obstetric background, the only issue of significance being a susceptibility to urinary infections.

Recurrent urinary tract infections are seen in 6% of women with sickle cell trait during pregnancy, with 16% showing microscopic hematuria.

169 A woman attends the antenatal clinic in a wheel chair with a known long-term traumatic spinal cord injury.

At what level of spinal injury and above would you be concerned about the occurrence of autonomic dysreflexia?

A. T6

B. T10

C. T12

D. L3

E. L5

TOG Article

Dawood R, Altanis E, Ribes-Pastor P, Ashworth F. Pregnancy and spinal cord injury. The Obstetrician & Gynaecologist 2014;16:99–107.

A spinal cord injury at the level of T6 or above results in the loss of supra-spinal control of the greater splanchnic sympathetic outflow. Autonomic dysreflexia results from disconnection of the sympathetic nervous system from supra-spinal regulation, disabling the negative feedback loop. A noxious stimulus below the level of the spinal cord injury will result in an uncontrolled sympathetic outflow below the level of the lesion. This causes a rise in blood pressure and can be fatal.

170 A 25-year-old woman presents at 12 weeks gestation. Four years earlier she presented with a deep vein thrombosis after fracturing her femur and undergoing a major orthopaedic operation. Her thrombophilia screen result is negative, she has no family history of thrombosis and she has a body mass index of 23 kg/m^2.

What thromboprophylaxis should be offered to this woman?

A. 6 weeks of low molecular weight heparin postnatal

B. Aspirin antenatally and 6 week of low molecular weight heparin postnatal

C. Immediate treatment of low molecular weight heparin until 37 weeks of gestation

D. Immediate treatment of low molecular weight heparin until 6 weeks postpartum

E. Start low molecular weight heparin at 28 weeks until 6 weeks postpartum

GTG 37a Reducing the Risk of Venous Thromboembolism during Pregnancy and the Puerperium

In women in whom the original VTE was provoked by major surgery from which they have recovered and who have no other risk factors, thromboprophylaxis with LMWH can be withheld antenatally until 28 weeks provided no additional risk factors are present (in which case they should be offered LMWH). They require close surveillance for the development of other risk factors.

Module 10

Management of Labour

171 A 32-year-old gravida 2 Para 1 has been transferred from a midwifery-led unit for lack of progress in labour at 4 cm. Her previous baby weighed 3100 g and was a normal delivery at 38 weeks gestation. On admission, her observations are normal and the cardiotocography (CTG) was reassuring. The midwife who examined her has diagnosed a complete breech presentation and this is confirmed on scan. The woman is very keen to have a vaginal delivery and decision has been taken to allow labour to continue. After 2 hours, there is no progress in labour and the CTG has become suspicious.

What is the most appropriate action?

A. Advise emergency caesarean section

B. Augment labour with syntocinon

C. Continue observation for one hour

D. Discuss ECV with the mother

E. Perform fetal blood sampling

GTG 20b The Management of Breech Presentation

Some women will choose a vaginal delivery with a breech presentation and diagnosis of breech in labour is not a contraindication to vaginal birth. Presentation should be frank or complete breech. While induction may be considered, labour augmentation is not recommended. While it is possible to obtain accurate acid–base values from the buttocks, given the small sample size of the study, it is not advised. Therefore, emergency caesarean section is the best option.

172 A Gravida 4 Para 3 (three normal deliveries at term) is admitted in preterm labour at 36 + 5 days. She is known to have polyhydramnios but relevant antenatal investigations have been normal.

Part 2 MRCOG: Single Best Answer Questions, First Edition.
Andrew Sizer, Chandrika Balachandar, Nibedan Biswas, Richard Foon, Anthony Griffiths, Sheena Hodgett, Banchhita Sahu and Martyn Underwood.
© 2016 John Wiley & Sons, Ltd. Published 2016 by John Wiley & Sons, Ltd.

An ultrasound scan at 36 weeks gestation had revealed the estimated fetal weight to be just below the 10th centile on a customized growth chart.

On examination, the cervix was 4 cm dilated with intact membranes and a high presenting part. Five minutes after admission there is spontaneous rupture of membranes and the CTG shows fetal bradycardia.

What needs to be excluded by a prompt vaginal examination?

A. Amniotic fluid embolism
B. Breech presentation
C. Cord prolapse
D. Placental abruption
E. Shoulder/arm prolapse

GTG 50 Umbilical Cord Prolapse

Cord prolapse should be suspected if there is fetal bradycardia or variable decelerations soon after membrane rupture – spontaneous or artificial. Multiparity, polyhydramnios, prematurity and SGA fetus with a high head in labour are all risk factors for cord prolapse. Perinatal mortality rate of 91/1000 has been reported with cord prolapse.

173 A primigravida who is a Type 1 diabetic is admitted in labour at 37 + 2 weeks gestation. The midwife has commenced sliding scale insulin infusion.

Between which values should the capillary blood glucose be maintained during labour?

A. 3 and 8 mmol/l
B. 3.5 and 5.9 mmol/l
C. 4 and 7 mmol/l
D. 5 and 9 mmol/l
E. 6 and 8 mmol/l

NICE NG3 Diabetes in Pregnancy

Monitor capillary plasma glucose every hour during labour and birth in women with diabetes, and ensure that it is maintained between 4 and 7 mmol/l.

174 A gravida 3 Para 2 (both full term normal deliveries) is admitted at term with confirmed rupture of membranes and labour has been augmented with syntocinon. The woman has suffered from recurrent herpes during pregnancy and is noted to have recurrent genital lesions on admission. At 4–5 cm dilatation, the liquor is noted to have grade II meconium and the CTG has been suspicious for the last 40 minutes.

What is the most appropriate action at this stage?

A. To advise emergency caesarean section to expedite delivery
B. To commence intravenous acyclovir
C. **To perform fetal blood sample to assess the acid base status of the baby**
D. To review the syntocinon and increase the dose to expedite delivery
E. To stop the syntocinon and advice to continue observation

BASHH RCOG Guideline Management of Genital Herpes in Pregnancy

It has been reported that invasive procedures (fetal blood sampling (FBS), application of fetal scalp electrodes, artificial rupture of membranes and/or instrumental deliveries) increase the risk of neonatal HSV infection. However, given the small background risk (0–3%) of transmission in this group, the increased risk associated with invasive procedures is unlikely to be clinically significant, and so may be used if required.

175 You are working in an Obstetric unit with level 2 Neonatal care facilities. A primigravida is admitted to the delivery suite at 32 weeks gestation with painful contractions and confirmed preterm prelabour rupture of membranes (PROM). She is pyrexial with a temperature of 38 °C and a pulse of 108/minute. CTG confirms regular contractions and there is fetal tachycardia of 170 bpm with good variability. A speculum examination had shown the cervix to be 2–3 cm dilated. Two weeks prior to this admission the woman had been seen in the day assessment unit with threatened preterm labour and had received two doses of dexamethasone.

What is the most appropriate management?

A. **Commence antibiotics after septic screen and allow labour to continue with continuous electronic fetal monitoring and inform neonatal unit**
B. Commence antibiotics and arrange in utero transfer to a level 3 neonatal unit
C. Commence tocolysis and arrange in utero transfer to a level 3 neonatal unit
D. Repeat dexamethasone, along with tocolysis and inform neonatal unit
E. Repeat dexamethasone, commence antibiotics and prepare for emergency caesarean section

GTG 1b Tocolysis for Women in Preterm Labour

Tocolysis is only considered for women with suspected preterm labour who have had an otherwise uncomplicated pregnancy and women likely to benefit most from tocolysis are those who are in very preterm labour, needing transfer to a hospital that can provide neonatal intensive care and those who have not yet completed a full course of corticosteroids. A Level 2 unit should be able to accept a baby at 32 weeks when the mother and the baby in question are not particularly suitable for transfer. Tocolysis should not be used where there is a contraindication to prolonging pregnancy – such as possible sepsis in the given scenario.

176 What type of headache is associated with a dural puncture?

    A. Fronto–occipital location

    B. Occipital location

    C. Temporal location

    D. Temporal with non-focal neurology

    E. Thunderclap

TOG Article

Revell K, Morrish P. Headaches in pregnancy. The Obstetrician & Gynaecologist 2014;16:179–184.

Puncture of the dura occurs in 0.5–2.5% of epidurals. If accidental dural puncture occurs with an epidural needle there is a 70–80% chance of a postdural puncture headache. The headache is usually in the fronto-occipital regions and radiates to the neck. It is characteristically worse on standing and typically develops 24–48 hours postpuncture. Conservative management includes hydration and simple analgesics.

Untreated, the headache typically lasts for 7–10 days but can last up to 6 weeks.

Epidural blood patch has a 60–90% cure rate.

177 A 24-year-old with a known hypersensitivity reaction to penicillin presents at 36 weeks of gestation in established labour. A high vaginal swab in this pregnancy has noted a growth of group B streptococcus. What intrapartum antibiotic prophylaxis would you offer?

    A. Benzyl penicillin

    B. Ceftriaxone

    C. Clindamycin

    D. Co-amoxiclav

    E. Erythromycin

TOG Article

Mugglestone MA, Murphy MS, Visintin C, Howe DT, Turner MA. Antibiotics for early-onset neonatal infection: a summary of the NICE guideline 2012. The Obstetrician & Gynaecologist 2014;16:87–92.

She has two known risk factors for early onset group B streptococcus neonatal infection namely maternal group B streptococcal colonisation, bacteriuria or infection in the current pregnancy, and also a preterm birth following spontaneous labour (before 37 weeks of gestation).

Other potential risk factors include suspected or confirmed rupture of membranes for more than18 hours in a preterm birth, intrapartum fever higher than 38 °C or confirmed or suspected chorioamnionitis or suspected or confirmed infection in another baby in the case of a multiple pregnancy.

Benzylpenicillin would not be suitable for all women (e.g., those allergic to penicillin), the recommended alternative to benzylpenicillin is clindamycin unless microbiological surveillance data reveal local bacterial resistance patterns indicating a different antibiotic.

178 A 25-year-old woman with no known drug allergies presents in early labour with ruptured membranes at 39 weeks gestation. She received intrapartum antibiotic prophylaxis (IAP) in her first labour following the identification of group B streptococcus (GBS) bacteriuria during pregnancy. She had a healthy baby with no neonatal problems. What is the most appropriate management?

  A. IAP with intravenous ampicillin
  B. IAP with intravenous benzylpenicillin
  C. IAP with intravenous clindamycin
  D. IAP with intravenous erythromycin
  E. No intrapartum antibiotic prophylaxis

TOG Article

Mugglestone M, Murphy M, Visintin C, Howe D, Turner M. Antibiotics for early-onset neonatal infection: a summary of the NICE guideline 2012. The Obstetrician and Gynaecologist 2014;16:87–92.

Another recommendation of relevance to obstetric practice is that pregnant women who have had GBS colonisation in a previous pregnancy but without infection in the baby should be reassured that this will not affect the management of the birth in the current pregnancy.

179 When considering local regimens for intrapartum antibiotic prophylaxis (IAP), what proportion of neonatal infection developing within 48 hours of birth in the United Kingdom is caused by group B streptococcus (GBS)?

A. 30%

B. 40%

C. 50%

D. 60%

E. 70%

TOG Article

Mugglestone M, Murphy M, Visintin C, Howe D, Turner M. Antibiotics for early-onset neonatal infection: a summary of the NICE guideline 2012. The Obstetrician and Gynaecologist 2014;16:87–92.

Two UK population-based surveillance studies on neonatal infection, both of which defined early onset neonatal infection as infection with onset within 48 hours of birth showed that after exclusion of coagulase negative staphylococci, which are usually considered to be blood sample contaminants soon after birth, the common organizms were Gram-positive in about 75% of cases. These included GBS (50% of cases), non-pyogenic streptococci and Staphylococcus aureus.

180 A 34-year-old woman presents in spontaneous labour at 38 weeks gestation in her second pregnancy, having had a previous prelabour caesarean section for breech presentation. In the first stage of labour, she develops continuous lower abdominal pain and a tachycardia. The fetal heart rate becomes bradycardic. She is delivered by urgent (category1) caesarean section and uterine rupture is confirmed. What is the risk of perinatal mortality?

A. 0.2%

B. 0.5%

C. 1%

D. 2%

E. 5%

TOG Article

Manoharan M, Wuntakal R, Erskine K. Uterine rupture: a revisit. The Obstetrician & Gynaecologist 2010;12:223–230.

A review of the literature found that 5% of symptomatic uterine ruptures were associated with perinatal mortality.

181 A 42-year-old woman is 39 weeks gestation in her second pregnancy having had a prior emergency caesarean section for fetal distress three years earlier. She is keen to give birth vaginally but is requesting induction of labour because of concerns regarding the increased risk of perinatal mortality associated with her age. What is the most appropriate method of induction to minimise the risk of uterine rupture in labour?

A. Amniotomy and oxytocin
B. Dinoprostone
C. Misoprostol
D. Oxytocin alone
E. Transcervical Foley catheter

TOG Article

Manoharan M, Wuntakal R, Erskine K. Uterine rupture: a revisit. The Obstetrician & Gynaecologist 2010;12:223–230.

Use of misoprostol as an induction agent in women with a previous scar is associated with an increased risk of uterine rupture of 5.6%. Unlike prostaglandins or oxytocin, cervical ripening with transcervical Foley catheters in women with previous caesarean delivery is not associated with increased risk of uterine rupture.

182 What is the incidence of cord prolapse with breech presentation?

A. 0.1%
B. 0.2%
C. 0.6%
D. 1%
E. 2%

GTG 50 Umbilical Cord Prolapse

The overall incidence of cord prolapse ranges from 0.1% to 0.6%. In the case of breech presentation, the incidence is higher at 1%.

183 When umbilical cord prolapse occurs in the community setting, what is the increase in risk of perinatal mortality?

A. 2 times
B. 4 times
C. 6 times
D. 8 times
E. 10 times

GTG 50 Umbilical Cord Prolapse

Perinatal mortality is increased by more than ten-fold when cord prolapse occurs outside the hospital compared to inside the hospital and neonatal morbidity is also increased in this circumstance.

184 In otherwise uncomplicated preterm labour, evidence suggests that use of tocolysis delays delivery by how long?
  A. 24 hours
  B. 48 hours
  C. 72 hours
  D. 7 days
  E. 14 days

GTG 1b Tocolysis for Women in Preterm Labour

Use of a tocolytic drug is associated with a prolongation of pregnancy for up to 7 days but with no significant effect on preterm birth and no clear effect on perinatal or neonatal morbidity.

185 Which tocolytic drug is comparably effective and has a similar incidence of maternal side effects to Atosiban when used to suppress preterm labour?
  A. Glyceryl trinitrate
  B. Indomethacin
  C. Magnesium sulphate
  D. Nifedipine
  E. Terbutaline

GTG 1b Tocolysis for Women in Preterm Labour

Nifedipine and Atosiban have comparable effectiveness in delaying birth for up to seven days. Nifedipine, atosiban and the COX inhibitors have fewer types of adverse effects and they occur less frequently than for beta-agonists but how they compare with each other is unclear.

186 A 25-year-old woman with no known drug allergies presents in early labour at 37 weeks gestation in her first pregnancy. Her membranes ruptured an hour prior to admission. Her temperature is 38.1 °C, she is clinically well and the fetal heart rate is normal. What is the most appropriate management?
  A. Category 1 caesarean section
  B. Category 2 caesarean section
  C. Treatment with intravenous antibiotics including benzylpenicillin
  D. Treatment with intravenous antibiotics including erythromycin
  E. Treatment with intravenous paracetamol and rechecking temperature in 2 hours

GTG 36 The Prevention of Early Onset Neonatal Group B Streptococcal Disease

Women who are pyrexial in labour should be offered broad-spectrum antibiotics including an antibiotic for prevention of neonatal (early onset Group B Streptococcus) EOGBS disease. Intrapartum pyrexia (>38 °C) is associated with a risk of EOGBS disease of 5.3/1000 (versus a background risk of 0.5/1000). In view of this increased risk, IAP should be offered in the presence of maternal pyrexia.

187 A 20-year-old woman presents at 40 weeks gestation in her first pregnancy with irregular contractions, offensive vaginal discharge and reduced fetal movements. She has a temperature of 39.2 °C and a tachycardia. On examination, the cervix is effaced and 4 cm dilated and membranes are absent. The fetal heart rate is 170 bpm. Broad spectrum antibiotics are administered after taking blood cultures. What is the most appropriate subsequent management?

A. Augmentation of labour with oxytocin

B. Category 2 caesarean section with general anaesthesia (GA)

C. Category 2 caesarean section with spinal anaesthesia

D. Epidural analgesia and fetal blood sampling (FBS)

E. Reassess progress in 4 hours

GTG 64a Bacterial Sepsis in Pregnancy

The effects of maternal sepsis on fetal well-being include the direct effect of infection on the fetus, the effect of maternal illness/shock and the effect of maternal treatment. The risk of neonatal encephalopathy and cerebral palsy is increased in the presence of intrauterine infection.

Epidural/spinal anesthesia should be avoided in women with sepsis and a general anaesthetic will usually be required for caesarean section.

188 A 24-year-old woman with sickle cell disease is admitted for induction of labour at 38 weeks gestation in her first pregnancy that is otherwise uncomplicated. Three hours after commencement of intravenous oxytocin, her oxygen saturation drops to 93%. What is the most appropriate immediate management?

A. Administer oxygen therapy and check arterial blood gases

B. Administer oxygen therapy and intravenous antibiotics

C. Category 1 caesarean section with general anesthesia (GA)

D. Category 2 caesarean section with regional analgesia

E. Stop the oxytocin infusion

GTG 61 Management of Sickle Cell Disease in Pregnancy

The demand for oxygen is increased during the intrapartum period and the use of pulse oximetry to detect hypoxia in the mother is appropriate during labour. Arterial blood gas analysis should be performed and oxygen therapy instituted if oxygen saturation is 94% or less.

Routine antibiotic prophylaxis in labour is currently not supported by evidence.

189 A 19-year-old woman is admitted at 34 weeks and 4 days gestation in her second pregnancy with spontaneous rupture of membranes and painful uterine contractions. Her first pregnancy resulted in a spontaneous preterm birth at 32 weeks gestation. On examination, the cervix is fully effaced and 6 cm dilated. What is the most appropriate treatment?

A. Atosiban 6.75 mg intravenously

B. Benzylpenicillin 1.2 g intravenously

C. Betamethasone 12 mg intramuscularly

D. Nifedipine 20 mg orally

E. Pethidine 100 mg intramuscularly

GTG 7 Antenatal Corticosteroids to Reduce Neonatal Morbidity

Clinicians should offer a single course of antenatal corticosteroids to women between 24 + 0 and 34 + 6 weeks of gestation who are at risk of preterm birth. Antenatal corticosteroid use reduces neonatal death within the first 24 hours and therefore should be given even if delivery is expected within this time.

190 A 31-year-old woman with well-controlled Type 1 diabetes is admitted for induction of labour at 38 weeks gestation in her second pregnancy having had a previous spontaneous normal birth at 36 weeks gestation. After vaginal examination confirms that she is 6 cm dilated, her blood sugar drops to 3.5 mmol/l and she has no symptoms of hypoglycemia.

What is the most appropriate management?

A. Allow light diet and recheck blood sugar after one hour

B. Commence intravenous dextrose and insulin infusion

C. Give intramuscular glucagon and recheck blood sugar after one hour

D. Give oral glucose gel and recheck blood sugar after one hour

E. Recheck blood sugar after 30 minutes

NICE NG3 Diabetes in Pregnancy: Management of Diabetes and Its Complications from Preconception to the Post Natal Period

Use intravenous dextrose and insulin infusion during labour and birth for women with diabetes whose capillary plasma glucose is not maintained between 4 and 7 mmol/l.

191 What percentage of women with PROM at term will go into labour within the next 24 hours?

A. 40%
B. 50%
C. 60%
D. 70%
E. 75%

NICE CG 190 Intrapartum Care: Care of Healthy Women and Their Babies During Childbirth

Sixty percent of women with prelabour rupture of the membranes will go into labour within 24 hours.

192 A low-risk 25-year-old woman at 40 weeks gestation is labouring in the birthing pool in her local midwifery-led unit. She is 8 cm dilated when her midwife checks the temperature of the water, which is 37.7 °C. What is the most appropriate immediate management?

A. Add cold water to the birthing pool
B. Ask her to get out of the pool temporarily
C. Encourage her to drink more water
D. Give oral paracetamol 1 g
E. Recheck the water temperature in 30 minutes

NICE CG 190 Intrapartum Care: Care of Healthy Women and Their Babies During Childbirth

For women labouring in water, monitor the temperature of the woman and the water hourly to ensure that the woman is comfortable and not becoming pyrexial. The temperature of the water should not be above 37.5 °C.

193 A low-risk 34-year-old woman in her second pregnancy is admitted in spontaneous labour at 39 weeks gestation. Her cervix is effaced and 5 cm dilated with membranes intact on admission.

She is examined again four hours later and is 6 cm dilated; she consents to artificial rupture of membranes (ARM), liquor is clear. What is the most appropriate method of fetal monitoring?

A. CTG for 20 minutes followed by intermittent auscultation

B. Continuous CTG with abdominal transducer

C. Continuous CTG with fetal scalp electrode

D. CTG for 40 minutes followed by intermittent auscultation

E. Intermittent auscultation

NICE CG 190 Intrapartum Care: Care of Healthy Women and Their Babies During Childbirth

Offer intermittent auscultation of the fetal heart rate to low-risk women in established first stage of labour in all birth settings.

Do not perform CTG for low-risk women in established labour.

Do not consider amniotomy alone for suspected delay in the established first stage of labour as an indication to start continuous CTG.

194 What proportion of intrapartum CTG with reduced fetal heart rate baseline variability and late decelerations results in moderate to severe cerebral palsy in children?

A. 0.1%

B. 0.2%

C. 0.5%

D. 1%

E. 1.5%

TOG Article

Sacco A, Muglu J, Navaratnarajah R, Hogg M. ST analysis for intrapartum fetal monitoring. The Obstetrician & Gynaecologist 2015; 17:5–12.

One study found that only 0.19% of children with intrapartum CTGs showing late decelerations and reduced variability had moderate or severe cerebral palsy, giving a false positive rate of 99.8%.

195 When evaluated as an adjunct to CTG for intrapartum fetal monitoring, of which outcome has STAN (ST analysis) been shown to reduce incidence?

A. Caesarean section

B. Low Apgar scores

C. Neonatal encephalopathy

D. Operative vaginal delivery

E. Severe fetal metabolic acidosis

TOG Article

Sacco A, Muglu J, Navaratnarajah R, Hogg M. ST analysis for intra-partum fetal monitoring. The Obstetrician and Gynaecologist 2015; 17:5–12.

The use of STAN was found to make no significant difference to births by caesarean section, the rate of severe fetal metabolic acidosis or the number of babies with neonatal encephalopathy. There was also no significant difference in the number of babies with low Apgar scores at 5 minutes or babies requiring neonatal intubation. The Cochrane review did find that the use of STAN resulted in fewer fetal scalp samples and fewer operative vaginal deliveries.

Module 11

Management of Delivery

196 What is the risk of neonatal herpes infection in a woman with recurrent genital HSV infection if lesions are present at the time of vaginal delivery?
A. 0–3%
B. 10–13%
C. 20–23%
D. 30–33%
E. 40–43%

BASHH RCOG Guideline Management of Genital Herpes in Pregnancy

Women with recurrent genital herpes should be informed that the risk of neonatal herpes is low, even if lesions are present at the time of delivery (0–3% for vaginal delivery). Vaginal delivery should be anticipated in the absence of other obstetric indications for a caesarean section.

197 A primigravida is in spontaneous preterm labour at 35 + 1 weeks of gestation. She has progressed satisfactorily in labour and has been pushing for ten minutes. Fifteen minutes prior to pushing, a fetal blood sampling had been performed due to a suspicious CTG and the result was normal. You have been asked to attend as the CTG shows prolonged bradycardia. You are not able to feel the fetal head abdominally and the vertex is at +2 station and is less than 45° from the occipito-anterior position.
What is the most appropriate course of action?
A. Expedite delivery by performing a caesarean section
B. Expedite delivery with low mid-cavity forceps
C. Expedite delivery with rotational forceps
D. Expedite delivery with Ventouse
E. Repeat fetal blood sampling

Part 2 MRCOG: Single Best Answer Questions, First Edition.
Andrew Sizer, Chandrika Balachandar, Nibedan Biswas, Richard Foon, Anthony Griffiths, Sheena Hodgett, Banchhita Sahu and Martyn Underwood.
© 2016 John Wiley & Sons, Ltd. Published 2016 by John Wiley & Sons, Ltd.

GTG 26 Operative Vaginal Delivery

Presenting part is considered 'low' if the leading part is +2 cm and not palpable abdominally. Thus, it is suitable for operative vaginal delivery. Vacuum extractor should not be used for gestation under 34 + 0 weeks due to increased risk of subgaleal and intracranial haemorrhage. Extreme caution is also advised for vacuum extraction between 34 + 0 and 36 + 0 weeks and best avoided if fetal blood sampling has been performed less than 30 minutes prior to the decision. Therefore, a low mid-cavity forceps is the best course of action.

198 A gravida 3 Para 2 is diagnosed with anterior placenta reaching to the os at 20 weeks gestation. She has had 2 previous caesarean sections. Further imaging with colour flow doppler at 32 weeks has confirmed major placenta praevia and placenta accreta.
What would be the recommendation for delivery?
A. Category 3 caesarean section as soon as possible
B. Elective caesarean section at 36–37 weeks
C. Elective caesarean section at 38 weeks
D. Elective caesarean section at 39 weeks
E. Elective caesarean section at term

GTG 27 Placenta Praevia, Placenta Accreta and Vasa Praevia: Diagnosis and Management

About 40% of the women with major placenta praevia and placenta accreta will deliver before 38 weeks. While delivery at 32 weeks will prevent it, there is a high risk of iatrogenic prematurity. Those with uncomplicated placenta praevia can be delivered at 38 weeks; those with placenta accreta are best delivered at 36–37 weeks following steroids for fetal lung maturity.

199 Sequential use of instruments increases neonatal trauma.
By what factor is the incidence of subdural and intracranial haemorrhage increased in this situation?
A. 1.5 times
B. 2–3 times
C. 3–4 times
D. Up to 5 times
E. 10 times

GTG 26 Operative Vaginal Delivery

While the rate of neonatal injuries is comparable between vacuum (1:860), forceps (1:664) and caesarean section during labour (1:954), the risk is increased significantly among babies exposed to sequential instrumentation with vacuum and forceps (1:256).

200 An emergency buzzer has been activated for shoulder dystocia. You are instructing two junior midwives to assist you in delivery with McRoberts' maneuvre.
What would you ask them to do?
A. Hyperflex and adduct maternal thighs onto her abdomen
B. Hyperflex and adduct maternal thighs on her abdomen
C. Perform an episiotomy
D. Place the mother in a lithotomy position
E. Provide fundal pressure

GTG 42 Shoulder Dystocia

Fundal pressure should not be used in shoulder dystocia as it can result in uterine rupture. Episiotomy may be necessary but only to allow internal vaginal maneuvres. McRoberts' maneuvre demands hyper-flexion and adduction of maternal thighs over her abdomen. This increases the relative anteroposterior diameter of the pelvic inlet by straightening the lumbo-sacral angle and rotating the maternal pelvis towards the head.

201 The hospital blood transfusion committee requires guidance with regard to the use of cell salvage in Obstetrics.
On which occasions of caesarean section is cell salvage recommended?
A. Only for women who reject the use of blood products
B. When the intra-operative blood loss is anticipated to be greater than 1000 ml
C. When the intra-operative blood loss is anticipated to be greater than 1500 ml
D. When there is a high risk of platelet dysfunction
E. When there is an established coagulopathy

GTG 47 Blood Transfusion in Obstetrics

Cell salvage is recommended for women in whom an intra-operative blood loss of more than 1500 ml is anticipated.

Cell salvage should only be used by health-care teams who use it regularly and have the necessary expertise and experience. Consent should be obtained and its use in obstetric patients should be subject to audit and monitoring.

202 In the case of a massive obstetric haemorrhage, above what level should fibrinogen be maintained?

A. 0.5 g/l

B. 1 g/l

C. 2 g/l

D. 5 g/l

E. 10 g/l

GTG 47 Blood Transfusion in Obstetrics

Fibrinogen levels should be maintained above 1.0 g/l by the use of FFP as above or two pools of Cryoprecipitate.

203 You are asked to assess a woman's perineum after a vaginal delivery. There is an extensive tear disrupting the superficial muscle and 70 % of the external anal sphincter. There is no disruption of the internal anal sphincter. How would you classify this perineal trauma?

A. Second degree tear

B. 3a tear

C. 3b tear

D. 3c tear

E. Fourth degree tear

GTG 29 The Management of Third and Fourth Degree Vaginal Tears

The following classification described by Sultan, has been adopted by the International Consultation on Incontinence and the RCOG.

First degree Injury to perineal skin only.

Second degree Injury to perineum involving perineal muscles but not involving the anal sphincter.

Third degree Injury to perineum involving the anal sphincter complex:

3a: Less than 50% of EAS thickness torn.

3b: More than 50% of EAS thickness torn.

3c: Both EAS and IAS torn.

Fourth degree Injury to perineum involving the anal sphincter complex (EAS and IAS) and anal epithelium.

204 A 40-year-old woman is diagnosed with acute myocardial infarction (AMI) at 36 weeks gestation in her second pregnancy, she is clinically stable. She had a previous normal vaginal delivery at term in her local hospital.

What is the most appropriate plan for timing and mode of delivery?

A. Antenatal steroids and delivery by elective caesarean section in her local hospital

B. Await spontaneous labour and delivery in her local hospital

C. Immediate transfer to a high risk obstetric unit and urgent delivery by caesarean section

D. Induction of labour at 38–39 weeks gestation in a high risk obstetric unit with intensive care expertise

E. Induction of labour in her local hospital at 37 weeks gestation

TOG Article

Wuntakal R, Shetty N, Ioannou E, Sharma S, Kurian J. Myocardial infarction in pregnancy. The Obstetrician & Gynaecologist 2013; 15:247–255.

If possible, delivery should be delayed by 2–3 weeks because of the increased risk of maternal mortality during this time. Delivery should take place in high risk obstetric units with intensive care expertise. The mode of delivery (vaginal or elective caesarean section) is based on obstetric and maternal factors as neither is associated with higher mortality.

205 A 28-year-old woman presents in spontaneous labour at 41 weeks gestation with a cephalic presentation in her third pregnancy having had two previous normal births. At the onset of the second stage, she ruptures her membranes and the fetal heart rate decelerates. Vaginal examination confirms umbilical cord prolapse with the fetal head in direct occipito-anterior position below the level of the ischial spines.

What is the optimal management?

A. Anticipation of normal delivery and encouragement to push

B. Bladder filling to displace the fetal head and replacement of the prolapsed umbilical cord

C. Category 1 caesarean section under general anaesthesia

D. Digital elevation of the fetal head and category 2 caesarean section with regional anaesthesia

E. Immediate operative vaginal delivery with ventouse extraction

GTG 50 Umbilical Cord Prolapse

Vaginal birth, in most cases operative, can be attempted at full dilatation if it is anticipated that birth would be accomplished quickly and safely, using standard techniques and taking care to avoid impingement of the cord when possible.

206 A 40-year-old woman with Type 2 diabetes is admitted for induction of labour at 38 weeks gestation in her third pregnancy having had two previous spontaneous normal births. She has epidural analgesia for pain relief and her labour is uncomplicated until shoulder dystocia is diagnosed after delivery of the fetal head. Additional help is summoned but the shoulders cannot be delivered with axial traction and suprapubic pressure in McRoberts' position.

What is the most appropriate subsequent management?

A. Adopt 'all fours' position

B. Attempt delivery of the posterior arm

C. Attempt Zavanelli maneuvre

D. Downward traction

E. Fundal pressure

GTG 42 Shoulder Dystocia

Internal maneuvres or 'all-fours' position should be used if the McRoberts' maneuvre and suprapubic pressure fail.

For a less mobile woman with epidural anaesthesia in place, internal maneuvres are more appropriate.

207 A low-risk 27-year-old woman is induced at 41+ 5 weeks gestation in her second pregnancy, having had a previous ventouse delivery for fetal distress. She has epidural analgesia for pain relief in labour. Following confirmation of full cervical dilatation and an hour of passive second stage, she pushes with contractions for 90 minutes without signs of imminent birth. She feels well, her contractions are strong, 4 in 10 minutes and the fetal heart rate is normal.

What is the most appropriate management?

A. Commence intravenous oxytocin

B. Consider operative vaginal delivery after a further 30 minutes, if no change

C. Consider operative vaginal delivery after a further 60 minutes, if no change

D. Discuss operative vaginal delivery immediately

E. Encourage directed pushing in lithotomy position

NICE CG 190 Intrapartum Care: Care of Healthy Women and Their Babies During Childbirth

Upon confirmation of full cervical dilatation in a woman with regional analgesia, unless the woman has an urge to push or the baby's head is visible, pushing should be delayed for at least 1 hour and longer if the woman wishes, after which she should be actively encouraged to push during contractions.

After diagnosis of full dilatation in a woman with regional analgesia, agree a plan with the woman in order to ensure that birth will have occurred within 4 hours regardless of parity.

208 Following a prolonged second stage of labour, a primigravida at term is examined in order to make a decision about operative vaginal delivery.

Abdominal examination indicates that the fetal head is not palpable.

Vaginal examination shows the presenting part to be in a direct occipito-anterior position with a station of +3, and a decision is made to perform a ventouse (vacuum extraction) delivery.

How would you classify this operative vaginal delivery?

A. High

B. Low – rotation of 45° or less

C. Low – rotation of more than 45°

D. Mid

E. Outlet

GTG 26 Operative Vaginal Delivery

Table 1. Classification for operative vaginal delivery

Outlet	Fetal scalp visible without separating the labia
	Fetal skull has reached the pelvic floor
	Sagittal suture is in the anterio-posterior diameter or right or left occiput anterior or posterior position (rotation does not exceed 45°)
	Fetal head is at or on the perineum
Low	Leading point of the skull (not caput) is at station plus 2 cm or more and not on the pelvic floor
	Two subdivisions:
	• rotation of 45° or less from the occipito-anterior position
	• rotation of more than 45° including the occipito-posterior position
Mid	Fetal head is no more than 1/5th palpable per abdomen
	Leading point of the skull is above station plus 2 cm but not above the ischial spines
	Two subdivisions:
	• rotation of 45° or less from the occipito-anterior position
	• rotation of more than 45° including the occipito-posterior position
High	Not included in the classification as operative vaginal delivery is not recommended in this situation where the head is 2/5th or more palpable abdominally and the presenting part is above the level of the ischial spines

Adapted from the American College of Obstetrics and Gynecology, 2000[23]

209 What is the lower limit of gestational age for the use of the vacuum extractor (ventouse)?

A. 32/40

B. 34/40

C. 36/40

D. 38/40

E. 40/40

GTG 26 Operative Vaginal Delivery

A vacuum extractor should not be used at gestations of less than 34 weeks +0 days. The safety of vacuum extraction at between 34 weeks +0 days and 36 weeks +0 days of gestation is uncertain and should therefore be used with caution.

210 What type of morbidity is <u>less</u> likely to be associated with vacuum extraction than with forceps delivery?

A. Cephalohematoma

B. Low Apgar score at 5 minutes

C. Neonatal jaundice

D. Retinal haemorrhage

E. Vaginal and perineal trauma

GTG 26 Operative Vaginal Delivery

Vacuum extraction compared with forceps is:
- more likely to fail delivery with the selected instrument (OR 1.7; 95% CI 1.3–2.2)
- more likely to be associated with cephalhaematoma (OR 2.4; 95% CI 1.7–3.4)
- more likely to be associated with retinal haemorrhage (OR 2.0; 95% CI 1.3–3.0)
- more likely to be associated with maternal worries about baby (OR 2.2; 95% CI 1.2–3.9)
- less likely to be associated with significant maternal perineal and vaginal trauma (OR 0.4; 95% CI 0.3–0.5)
- no more likely to be associated with delivery by caesarean section (OR 0.6; 95% CI 0.3–1.0)
- no more likely to be associated with low 5-minute Apgar scores (OR 1.7; 95% CI 1.0–2.8)
- no more likely to be associated with the need for phototherapy (OR 1.1; 95% CI 0.7–1.8).

Module 12

Postnatal Care

211 A 38-year-old Asian mother has delivered her fourth baby normally. She is a known Type 2 diabetic and was taking Metformin prior to pregnancy for glycemic control. From 32 weeks gestation, Isophane insulin was added twice daily in addition to Metformin to achieve glycemic control. The woman is planning to breast feed.

What advise should be given with regard to a hypoglycemic agent in the postnatal period?

A. Continue all the medications for the first 24 hours after delivery and then resume Metformin as per prepregnancy with monitoring of blood sugar

B. Stop all medications and follow diet control with monitoring of blood sugar

C. Stop Insulin and advise Metformin as per prepregnancy with monitoring of blood sugar

D. Stop Metformin and continue Isophane insulin twice daily until breast feeding has stopped

E. Stop Metformin and continue Isophane insulin at half the dose used during pregnancy until breastfeeding is stopped

NICE NG3 Diabetes in Pregnancy

Diabetic mothers are at increased risk of hypoglycemia in the postnatal period as their insulin requirements drop immediately after birth. Gestational diabetics who needed insulin during pregnancy should be advised to stop all the insulin immediately after birth. Type 1 and 2 diabetics should be able to go back to their regime as per prepregnancy. Metformin is safe and can be resumed by mothers who choose to breast-feed immediately after birth.

Part 2 MRCOG: Single Best Answer Questions, First Edition.
Andrew Sizer, Chandrika Balachandar, Nibedan Biswas, Richard Foon,
Anthony Griffiths, Sheena Hodgett, Banchhita Sahu and Martyn Underwood.
© 2016 John Wiley & Sons, Ltd. Published 2016 by John Wiley & Sons, Ltd.

212 A 17-year-old Para 1 is attending for postnatal follow-up 6 weeks after an emergency caesarean section for severe pre-eclampsia and HELLP at 27+ 2 days gestation. The baby was severely growth-restricted and is still in the neonatal unit.

What is her risk of pre-eclampsia in a future pregnancy?

A. 13%

B. 16%

C. 25%

D. 45%

E. 55%

NICE CG107 Hypertension in Pregnancy

Recurrence rate of gestational hypertension varies from 1:8 (13%) to 1:2 (53%). Chance of pre-eclampsia in future pregnancy is about 1:6 (16%) However, it increases to 1:4 (25%) if it was severe and associated with eclampsia or HELLP requiring delivery before 34 weeks and to 1:2 (55%) if the delivery was before 28 weeks.

213 A woman who is a recent immigrant to the United Kingdom is admitted in labour and delivers rapidly. At delivery, the midwife had noted that the liquor was offensive and appropriate swabs were taken. The mother is also noted to have a low-grade pyrexia and mild tachycardia. Within minutes of antibiotic administration, the mother collapses and anaphylactic shock is diagnosed. An A, B, C, D, E approach has been initiated.

What is the definitive treatment for anaphylaxis?

A. 50 micrograms (0.5 ml) of intra-cardiac 1:10,000 adrenaline

B. 500 micrograms (0.5 ml) of 1:1000 adrenaline intramuscularly

C. 500 micrograms (0.5 ml) of 1:1000 adrenaline intravenously

D. Chlorpheneramine 10 mg intramuscularly

E. Hydrocortisone 200 mg – Intravenously

GTG 56 Maternal Collapse in Pregnancy and the Puerperium

The definitive treatment for anaphylaxis is 500 micrograms (0.5 ml) of 1:1000 adrenaline. This dose is for intramuscular use only. It can be repeated if there is no response after 5 minutes. Experienced clinicians might be able to use a bolus of 50 microgram (0.5 ml of 1:10,000 solution) intravenously. Chlorphenamine 10 mg and hydrocortisone 200 mg are adjuvant treatments and can be given intramuscularly or by slow intravenous injection.

214 A primigravida aged 30 attends the antenatal clinic for booking. She is known to have Bipolar Disorder and was taking lithium, which was stopped preconceptually due to concerns over fetal toxicity. Her mother is known to have bipolar disorder.

What is her risk of developing postpartum psychosis?

A. 25%

B. 35%

C. 40%

D. 50%

E. **70%**

TOG Article

Di Florio A, Smith S, Jones I. Postpartum psychosis. The Obstetrician & Gynaecologist 2013;15:145–50.

Women with bipolar disorder have at least a 1:4 risk of postpartum psychosis and need close review during perinatal period even if they are well. Those with a family history are at a higher risk with greater than 1 in 2 deliveries being affected by postpartum psychosis. Postpartum recurrence rate is 2.9 times higher than in nonpregnant women who stop medication for other reasons in the weeks between 41and 64 after stopping (70% vs 24%). Hormonal factors and sleep deprivation contribute to increased risk of recurrence following childbirth.

215 A 35-year-old grandmultipara has had a major postpartum haemorrhage (PPH) following a normal delivery. Mechanical and pharmacological measures have failed to control the bleeding. Examination has confirmed that there are no retained placental tissue in the uterine cavity and absence of trauma to genital tract.

What is the most appropriate first-line surgical management?

A. B-Lynch or modified compression sutures

B. **Balloon tamponade**

C. Ligation of internal iliac artery

D. Postpartum hysterectomy

E. Selective arterial embolisation

GTG 52 Prevention and Management of Postpartum Haemorrhage

Intrauterine balloon tamponade is the most appropriate first-line surgical intervention for most women if uterine atony is the main cause of haemorrhage.

216 Active management of the third stage of labour reduces the risk of PPH.

By what proportion is the risk of PPH reduced by prophylactic oxytocic agents?

A. 30%

B. 40%

C. 50%

D. 60%

E. 80%

GTG 52 Prevention and Management of Postpartum Haemorrhage

Prophylactic oxytocic should be offered routinely in the management of the third stage of labour in all women as they reduce the risk of PPH by about 60%. The prophylactic agent of choice in the third stage for women without risk factors for PPH delivering vaginally is oxytocin 5 or 10 iu by intramuscular injection. For women delivering by caesarean section, oxytocin 5 iu by slow intravenous injection is recommended to encourage contraction of the uterus and to decrease blood loss.

217 A 33-year-old multiparous woman has been taking therapeutic low molecular weight heparin (LMWH) from 34 weeks gestation for confirmed pulmonary embolism. She has an uncomplicated spontaneous normal vaginal delivery at 38 weeks gestation.

What is the most appropriate postnatal management?

A. Continue therapeutic LMWH for 14 days postnatally

B. Continue therapeutic LMWH for a total of 3 months from the time of commencement of treatment

C. Switch to oral anticoagulant 24 hours after delivery

D. Switch to prophylactic LMWH and continue for 6 weeks postnatally

E. Switch to prophylactic LMWH and continue for a total of 3 months from time of commencement of treatment

GTG 37b The Acute Management of Thrombosis and Embolism During Pregnancy and Puerperium

Women receiving therapeutic LMWH during pregnancy for confirmed thromboembolic disease should continue the therapeutic dose for at least 6 weeks postnatally and until a minimum of 3 months of treatment has been given in total since commencement of treatment. Oral anticoagulation can be offered but should be avoided until at least the fifth day.

218 A 37-year-old primigravida, 102 kg, and a BMI of 40 kg/m² is seen in the antenatal clinic for booking. She has conceived following a long period of subfertility through assisted conception. Ultrasound scan had confirmed a di-chorionic, di-amniotic twin pregnancy of 11+ 5 days gestation. Prophylactic LMWH had been given throughout pregnancy. A category 3 caesarean section had been performed at 37 weeks.

What is recommended as the best practice with regard to reducing maternal risk of VTE in the puerperium?

A. LMWH 20 mg per day for 6 weeks postnatally

B. LMWH 60 mg per day for 7 days postnatally

C. Prophylactic LMWH 60 mg per day for 6 weeks postnatally

D. TED stockings, mobilisation and hydration

E. Therapeutic LMWH for 7 days postnatally

GTG 37a Reducing Risk of Thrombosis and Embolism during Pregnancy and Puerperium

All women who undergo caesarean section should be considered for thromboprophylaxis with LMWH for at least 10 days after delivery. However, this is not required for women who undergo elective caesarean section if there are no other additional risk factors. Thromboprophylaxis should be continued for 6 weeks after delivery in high-risk women as the VTE risk persists for 6 weeks postpartum and a caesarean section continues to be a significant risk factor for fatal pulmonary embolism.

219 A 25-year-old woman goes into spontaneous labour at term. She has an undiagnosed Chlamydia infection. What is the chance that she will develop a puerperal infection if she delivers vaginally?

A. 5%

B. 10%

C. 14%

D. 34%

E. 44%

TOG Article

Allstaff S, Wilson J. The management of sexually transmitted infections in pregnancy. TOG 2012;14;25–32.

Up to 34% of women with chlamydia delivering vaginally will develop puerperal infection. Approximately, 50% of neonates born to women with untreated chlamydia will develop ophthalmia neonatorum and about 15% will develop chlamydia pneumonitis.

220 Chlamydia testing should be performed in women with lower genital tract symptoms and intrapartum or postpartum fever, and in mothers of infants with ophthalmia neonatorum.

When should the test of cure be done after initial treatment in pregnancy?

A. 1–2 weeks after completion of treatment
B. 3–4 weeks after completion of treatment
C. 5–6 weeks after completion of treatment
D. 7–8 weeks after completion of treatment
E. 9–10 weeks after completion of treatment

TOG Article

Allstaff S, Wilson J. The management of sexually transmitted infections in pregnancy. TOG 2012;14;25–32.

Women who have chlamydia treated in pregnancy are at increased risk of a subsequent test being positive because of treatment failure or reinfection; hence, the importance of public health interventions. A test of cure should be performed 5–6 weeks after completion of treatment and repeat screening in the third trimester is recommended.

221 In a breastfeeding population, what is the risk of mother to child transmission of HIV due to breastfeeding?

A. 0–4%
B. 5–14%
C. 24–44%
D. 45–64%
E. 66–85%

TOG Article

Byrne L, Fakoya A, Harding K. HIV in pregnancy. TOG 2012;14; 17–24.

Postnatal transmission of HIV occurs due to breastfeeding. Breast milk from HIV-infected mothers contains cell-free HIV RNA and intracellular HIV DNA and both are considered to contribute to transmission. In breastfeeding populations, 24–44% of all mother to child transmission of HIV is due to breastfeeding and the cumulative probability of HIV transmission is fairly constant over time and therefore correlates with the duration of breastfeeding.

222 What proportion of cases of neonatal Herpes simplex infection are due to HSV-2?

A. 10%

B. 20%

C. 30%

D. 40%

E. **50%**

BASHH RCOG Guideline Management of genital herpes in pregnancy

Neonatal herpes may be caused by herpes simplex virus type 1 (HSV-1) or herpes simplex virus type 2 (HSV-2) as either viral type can cause genital herpes in the mother. Approximately, 50% of neonatal herpes is due to HSV-1 and 50% due to HSV-2.

223 A woman with confirmed obstetric cholestatis has a normal vaginal delivery.

How long after delivery should repeat liver function tests be performed?

A. 48 hours

B. 5 days

C. 7 days

D. **10 days**

E. 6 weeks

GTG 43 Obstetric Cholestasis

Postnatally, LFTs should be deferred for at least 10 days.

Postnatal resolution of symptoms and of biochemical abnormalities is required to secure the diagnosis. In normal pregnancy, LFTs may increase in the first 10 days of the puerperium. In a pregnancy complicated by obstetric cholestasis, routine measurement of LFTs should be deferred beyond this time, and can be performed before the postnatal follow-up visit.

224 A woman in the second postpartum week presents with confusion, bewilderment, delusions and hallucinations. She feels hopeless and care of the baby has been affected.

What is the most likely diagnosis?

A. Baby blues

B. **Postpartum psychosis**

C. Severe pre-eclampsia

D. Severe sepsis

E. Substance abuse

TOG Article

Di Florio A, Smith S, Jones I. Postpartum psychosis. The Obstetrician & Gynaecologist 2013;15:145–50.

The distinctive clinical features of postpartum psychosis include sudden onset and rapid deterioration. The vast majority of episodes have their onset within 2 weeks of delivery, with over 50% of symptom onsets occurring on days 1–3. The clinical picture often changes rapidly, with wide fluctuations in the intensity of symptoms and severe swings of mood. Common symptoms and signs include:

- A wide variety of psychotic phenomena such as delusions and hallucinations, the content of which is often related to the new child.
- Affective (mood) symptoms, both elation and depression.
- Disturbance of consciousness marked by an apparent confusion, bewilderment or perplexity.

225 Mental disorders during pregnancy and the postnatal period can have serious consequences on the health of the mother and her baby. It is vital that these women be managed by the appropriate health-care professionals.

Which health-care professional(s) should care for pregnant women with a history of postpartum psychosis?

A. Community mental health team

B. Community midwife

C. General obstetrician

D. General practitioner

E. Specialised perinatal mental health service

RCOG GP 14 Management of Women with Mental Health Issues During Pregnancy and the Postnatal Period

Indications for referral to specialised perinatal mental health services, where available, otherwise general psychiatry services.

Women with current illness where there are symptoms of psychosis, severe anxiety, severe depression, suicidality, self-neglect, harm to others or significant interference with daily functioning. Such illnesses may include psychotic disorders, severe anxiety or depression, obsessive-compulsive disorder and eating disorders.

Women with a history of bipolar disorder or schizophrenia.

Women with previous serious postpartum mental illness (puerperal psychosis).

Women on complex psychotropic medication regimens.

226 Postpartum psychosis is a psychiatric emergency usually needing admission.

What is the incidence of postpartum psychosis in the general population?

A. 1 in 100 deliveries

B. 1 in 1000 deliveries

C. 1 in 10,000 deliveries

D. 1 in 100,000 deliveries

E. 1 in 1,000,000 deliveries

TOG Article

Di Florio A, Smith S, Jones I. Postpartum psychosis. The Obstetrician & Gynaecologist 2013;15:145–50.

Record-linkage studies estimate the admission rates to psychiatric hospital in the postpartum as about 1–2 per 1000 births in the general population.

227 A woman in the first postpartum week presents with mood swings ranging from elation to sadness, irritability, anxiety and decreased concentration. Care of the baby is not impaired and the woman does not feel suicidal.

What is the most likely diagnosis?

A. Baby blues

B. Postpartum psychosis

C. Severe pre-eclampsia

D. Severe sepsis

E. Substance abuse

TOG Article

Di Florio A, Smith S, Jones I. Postpartum psychosis. The Obstetrician & Gynaecologist 2013;15:145–50.

Baby blues affect 30–80% of birth and cause transient emotional liability during the first postpartum week. The mother typically presents mood swings ranging from elation to sadness, insomnia, tearfulness, crying spells, irritability, anxiety and decreased concentration. Care of the baby is not impaired, hopelessness and worthlessness are not prominent and women do not feel suicidal. It is self-limiting, but assessment should ensure that the woman is not and does not become more severely depressed.

228 At a woman's first contact with primary care or her booking visit and during the early postnatal period efforts should be made to ask about the woman's mental health and well-being using the 2 item GAD2 Scale:
What is the GAD-2 scale used for?
A. **Identification of anxiety**
B. Identification of bipolar disorder
C. Identification of depression
D. Risk of developing mania in pregnancy
E. Risk of puerperal psychosis

NICE CG 192 Antenatal and Postnatal Mental Health

The 2 item Generalised Anxiety Disorder scale (GAD2) is used to identify anxiety disorders in pregnancy.

During the past month, have you been feeling nervous, anxious or on edge?

During the past month have you not been able to stop or control worrying?

229 A woman with a history of severe depression presents with mild depression in pregnancy or the postnatal period.
What is the best plan of care?
A. Admit to mother and baby unit for further management
B. **Commence pharmacotherapy**
C. Consider ECT (Electro-convulsive therapy)
D. Offer CBT(Cognitive behaviour therapy)
E. Reassure and wait and watch

NICE CG 192 Antenatal and Postnatal Mental Health

For a woman with a history of severe depression who initially presents with mild depression in pregnancy or the postnatal period, consider a TCA\SSRI.

230 All health-care professionals providing assessment and interventions for mental health problems in pregnancy and the postnatal period should understand the variations in their presentation and course.
Along with this there should be knowledge of how these variations affect treatment, and the context in which they are assessed and treated (e.g., maternity services, health visiting and mental health services).

When a woman with a known or suspected mental health problem is referred in postnatal period within what time frame should assessment for treatment be initiated?

A. 2 weeks

B. 4 weeks

C. 6 weeks

D. 8 weeks

E. 10 weeks

NICE CG 192 Antenatal and Postnatal Mental Health

When a woman with a known or suspected mental health problem is referred in pregnancy or the postnatal period, assess for treatment within 2 weeks of referral and provide psychological interventions within 1 month of initial assessment.

Module 13

Gynaecological Problems

231 Following a spontaneous miscarriage at 8/40 gestation, a woman is referred to the gynaecology clinic with persistent irregular vaginal bleeding.

What initial investigation should be performed?

A. Endocervical swab to screen for chlamydia and gonorrhoea

B. Endometrial biopsy

C. Pelvic ultrasound scan

D. Serum βHCG level

E. Urinary pregnancy test

GTG 38 The Management of Gestational Trophoblastic Disease

Any woman who develops persistent vaginal bleeding after a pregnancy event is at risk of having gestational trophoblastic neoplasia (GTN).

A urine pregnancy test should be performed in all cases of persistent or irregular vaginal bleeding after a pregnancy event.

232 A 30-year-old woman attends the gynaecology clinic with discomfort in the left iliac fossa and clinical examination suggests a pelvic mass.

An ultrasound scan is arranged, which demonstrates a simple cyst in the left ovary with a diameter of 45 mm. The right ovary and uterus appear normal.

What other investigation is required?

A. Alfa-feto protein

B. CA-125

C. β-HCG

D. Lactate dehydrogenase

E. No investigation required

Part 2 MRCOG: Single Best Answer Questions, First Edition.
Andrew Sizer, Chandrika Balachandar, Nibedan Biswas, Richard Foon, Anthony Griffiths, Sheena Hodgett, Banchhita Sahu and Martyn Underwood.
© 2016 John Wiley & Sons, Ltd. Published 2016 by John Wiley & Sons, Ltd.

GTG 62 Management of Suspected Ovarian Masses in Premenopausal Women

Women with small (less than 50 mm diameter) simple ovarian cysts generally do not require follow-up as these cysts are very likely to be physiologic and almost always resolve within three menstrual cycles.

A serum CA-125 assay need not be undertaken in all premenopausal women when an ultrasonographic diagnosis of a simple ovarian cyst has been made.

Lactate dehydrogenase (LDH), α-FP and hCG should be measured in all women under age 40 with a complex ovarian mass because of the possibility of germ cell tumors.

233 A 40-year-old woman with BMI 32 kg/m^2 is referred to the gynae-cology clinic with secondary amenorrhoea. She has two children and her partner had a vasectomy 5 years ago.

An ultrasound scan is performed, which shows a normal uterus with endometrial thickness 6 mm.

Both ovaries have a typical polycystic appearance.

What would be the recommended management?

A. Endometrial biopsy

B. Induction of 3-monthly withdrawal bleeds with pro-gestagens

C. Metformin twice daily

D. Ovulation induction with clomiphene citrate

E. Reassure and discharge

GTG 33 Long-Term Consequences of Polycystic Ovary Syndrome

Oligo- or amenorrhoea in women with Polycystic Ovary Syndrome (PCOS) may predispose to endometrial hyperplasia and later carci-noma. It is good practice to recommend treatment with gestogens to induce a withdrawal bleed at least every 3 to 4 months.

Transvaginal ultrasound should be considered in the absence of with-drawal bleeds or abnormal uterine bleeding. In PCOS, an endometrial thickness of less than 7 mm is unlikely to be hyperplasia.

A thickened endometrium or an endometrial polyp should prompt consideration of endometrial biopsy and/or hysteroscopy.

234 A 55-year-old woman attends the gynaecology clinic. She is suffer-ing with terrible menopausal symptoms and cannot sleep because of the frequency of hot flushes.

She is requesting hormone replacement therapy (HRT) for symptom relief. She is currently healthy but has a history of a deep venous thrombosis in her calf following a fractured femur as a result of an accident 10 years ago.

Her last menstrual period was 2 years ago and her uterus is intact. What would you recommend?

A. All HRT is contraindicated in this situation

B. Oestrogen and testosterone implants

C. Oral continuous combined HRT

D. Raloxifene

E. Transdermal continuous combined HRT

GTG 19 Venous Thromboembolism and Hormone Replacement Therapy

A personal history of thrombosis is a contraindication to oral HRT. If it is observed that quality of life is so severely affected that the benefits of HRT outweigh the risks, a transdermal preparation should be used.

235 A woman opts to take oral continuous combined HRT for 5 years after the menopause.

In which year of HRT use will her risk of venous thromboembolism (VTE) be greatest?

A. 1st year

B. 2nd year

C. 3rd year

D. 4th year

E. 5th year

GTG 19 Venous Thromboembolism and Hormone Replacement Therapy

The risk of VTE is highest in the 1st year of HRT use, with no evidence of continuing risk on stopping HRT.

236 What is the karyotype of a woman with Mayer–Rokitansky–Kuster–Hauser (MRKH) syndrome (mullerian agenesis)?

A. 45 XO

B. 46 XX

C. 46 XY

D. 47 XXX

E. 47 XXY

TOG Article

Valappil S, Chetan U, Wood N, Garden A. Mayer–Rokitansky–Kuster–Hauser syndrome: diagnosis and management. The Obstetrician & Gynaecologist 2012;14:93–98.

Mayer–Rokitansky–Kuster–Hauser (MRKH) syndrome (mullerian agenesis) is a malformation complex characterised by congenital absence of the upper two-thirds of the vagina and an absent or rudimentary uterus in women who have normal development of secondary sexual characteristics and a 46 XX karyotype.

237 A 20-year-old girl attends the gynaecology clinic with her mother. She presents with primary amenorrhoea.

On examination she is tall with a BMI of 19 kg/m². She has normal breast development, but a short blind-ending vagina. There is no axillary or pubic hair.

What is the most likely diagnosis?

A. Complete androgen insensitivity syndrome

B. Klinefelter syndrome

C. Mullerian agenesis

D. Swyer syndrome

E. Turners syndrome

TOG Article

Valappil S, Chetan U, Wood N, Garden A. Mayer–Rokitansky–Kuster–Hauser syndrome: diagnosis and management. The Obstetrician & Gynaecologist 2012;14:93–98.

Complete androgen insensitivity syndrome (CAIS) can easily be mistaken for MRKH syndrome. In CAIS, the phenotype is female with a short, blind-ending vagina but the karyotype is 46 XY and the patient has no axillary or pubic hair.

238 A 48-year-old woman attends the gynaecology clinic complaining of heavy menstrual bleeding (HMB) and occasional intermenstrual bleeding.

Her haemoglobin level is 112 g/l.

An ultrasound scan demonstrated no obvious abnormality.

What other investigation is required?

A. Coagulation screen

B. Diagnostic hysteroscopy

C. Endometrial biopsy

D. MRI scan of pelvis

E. Serum FSH level

NICE CG 44 Heavy Menstrual Bleeding

If appropriate, a biopsy should be taken to exclude endometrial cancer or atypical hyperplasia. Indications for a biopsy include, for example, persistent intermenstrual bleeding, and, in women aged 45 and over, treatment failure or ineffective treatment.

239 A 42-year-old woman with oligomenorrhoea and hirsutism presents to the gynaecology clinic. She recently had a prolonged episode of vaginal bleeding, but an ultrasound scan and endometrial biopsy performed in primary care both reported normal results. She is obese with a BMI of 40 kg/m². She has mild hypertension but does not require antihypertensive therapy. She has no other medical problems.

Her father suffered from Type 2 Diabetes mellitus.

What further investigation is required?

A. LH:FSH ratio
B. MRI scan of pelvis
C. Oral glucose tolerance test
D. Pregnancy test
E. Serum cholesterol

GTG 33 Long-Term Consequences of Polycystic Ovary Syndrome

Women presenting with PCOS, particularly if they are obese (body mass index greater than 30), have a strong family history of Type 2 diabetes or are over the age of 40 years, are at increased risk of Type 2 diabetes and should be offered a glucose tolerance test.

240 A 35-year-old woman attends the gynaecology clinic complaining of worsening HMB.

Investigations have been performed in primary care. Her haemoglobin level is 123 g/l and a pelvic ultrasound scan showed no obvious abnormality.

What is the most appropriate first-line pharmacological treatment?

A. Combined oral contraceptive pill
B. Cyclical Norethisterone
C. Depo Medroxyprogesterone acetate
D. Levonorgestrel-containing intrauterine system
E. Tranexamic acid

NICE CG 44 Heavy Menstrual Bleeding

If history and investigations indicate that pharmaceutical treatment is appropriate and either hormonal or nonhormonal treatments are acceptable, treatments should be considered in the following order:

Levonorgestrel-releasing intrauterine system (LNG-IUS) provided long-term (at least 12 months) use is anticipated.

Tranexamic acid or non-steroidal anti-inflammatory drugs (NSAIDs) or combined oral contraceptives (COCs).

Norethisterone (15 mg) daily from days 5 to 26 of the menstrual cycle, or injected long-acting progestogens.

241 What percentage of women experience severe premenstrual symptoms?
   A. 1%
   B. 5%
   C. 10%
   D. 15%
   E. 20%

GTG 48 Management of Premenstrual Syndrome

Approximately 5% of women experience severe premenstrual symptoms, which include depression, anxiety, irritability and loss of confidence, as well as physical symptoms including bloating and mastalgia.

242 The aetiology of premenstrual syndrome (PMS) remains unclear but appears to be related to the effect of cyclical ovarian activity on neurotransmitters.
   Which neurotransmitters are considered to have a key role?
   A. Adrenaline and Dopamine
   B. Adrenaline and Noradrenaline
   C. Gamma-aminobutyric acid (GABA) and Noradrenaline
   D. Gamma-aminobutyric acid (GABA) and Serotonin
   E. Serotonin and Dopamine

GTG 48 Management of Premenstrual Syndrome

The precise aetiology of PMS remains unknown but cyclical ovarian activity and the effect of estradiol and progesterone on the neurotransmitters serotonin and gamma-aminobutyric acid (GABA) appear to be key factors.

243 A 70-year-old woman undergoes a dual-energy X-ray absorptiometry (DXA) scan to assess her bone mineral density.
What T score is diagnostic of osteoporosis?
A. +2.5
B. +1.0
C. −1.0
D. −2.5
E. −5.0

TOG Article

Kwun S, Laufgraben MJ, Gopalakrishnan G. Prevention and treatment of postmenopausal osteoporosis. The Obstetrician & Gynaecologist 2012;14:251–6.

Box 2. World Health Organization (WHO) bone mineral density (BMD) diagnostic criteria

Bone density category	WHO BMD diagnostic criteria[4]
Normal	T-score $\geq$ −1
Osteopenia	T score <−1 but >−2.5
Osteoporosis	T score $\leq$ −2.5
Established osteoporosis denotes patients who meet BMD criteria for diagnosis who have already experienced fragility fracture	

244 What is the mode of action of bisphosphonates?
A. Calcitonin antagonist
B. Decreased bone resorption
C. Increased bone formation
D. Inhibition of release of parathyroid hormone
E. Vitamin D agonist

TOG Article

Kwun S, Laufgraben MJ, Gopalakrishnan G. Prevention and treatment of postmenopausal osteoporosis. The Obstetrician & Gynaecologist 2012;14:251–6.

Bisphosphonates inhibit osteoclast-mediated bone resorption. By slowing the bone remodelling cycle, bisphosphonates increase BMD in postmenopausal women and reduce the risk of osteoporotic fractures.

245 What is the most common side effect of bisphosphonates?
  A. Diarrhoea and vomiting
  B. Flu-like illness
  C. Oesophageal irritation
  D. Osteonecrosis of the jaw
  E. Urinary frequency

TOG Article

Kwun S, Laufgraben MJ, Gopalakrishnan G. Prevention and treatment of postmenopausal osteoporosis. The Obstetrician & Gynaecologist 2012;14:251–6.

The most common side effect of bisphosphonates is oesophageal irritation. Therefore, individuals with oesophageal abnormalities who delay oesophageal emptying and those who cannot stand or sit upright for at least 30 to 60 minutes after dosing should not receive bisphosphonates.

246 Raloxifene is a selective oestrogen receptor modulator.
  What kind of action does this drug have on the endometrium, breast and bone?

| | Tissue | |
Endometrium	Bone	Breast
A. agonist	agonist	agonist
B. agonist	antagonist	antagonist
C. antagonist	**agonist**	**antagonist**
D. antagonist	antagonist	agonist
E. antagonist	antagonist	antagonist

TOG Article

Kearney C, Purdie D. Selective oestrogen receptor modulators (SERMS). The Obstetrician & Gynaecologist 2000,2:6–10.

Raloxifene is considered to act like oestrogen and to inhibit bone resorption and turnover.

In an analysis with a median follow-up of 40 months, raloxifene was shown to decrease the risk of developing an ER positive breast tumor by 90%.

No oestrogenic effects were seen in endometrial samples obtained from women taking raloxifene.

247 A 29-year-old woman presents with a constant ongoing pain in the pelvis.
  The pain does not occur exclusively with menstruation or intercourse and the woman is not pregnant.

For what minimum duration should the pain occur before it is deemed chronic?

A. 1 week

B. 1 month

C. 3 months

D. 6 months

E. 1 year

GTG 41 The Initial Management of Chronic Pelvic Pain

Chronic pelvic pain can be defined as intermittent or constant pain in the lower abdomen or pelvis of a woman for at least 6 months in duration, not occurring exclusively with menstruation or intercourse and not associated with pregnancy. It is a symptom not a diagnosis.

248 An 18-year-old girl presents with chronic lower abdominal pain. In what percentage of patients attending a gynaecology outpatient clinic with lower abdominal/pelvic pain would you expect to find irritable bowel syndrome (IBS)?

A. 10%

B. 25%

C. 33%

D. 50%

E. 66%

GTG 41 The Initial Management of Chronic Pelvic Pain

Symptoms suggestive of IBS or interstitial cystitis are often present in women with chronic pelvic pain.

In a study of 798 women attending a gynaecology clinic, 50% of women referred because of pain had symptoms suggestive of IBS.

249 A 24-year-old girl attends the gynaecology clinic with persistent pain over her Pfannenstiel scar that has not settled since her caesarean section of 6 months.

What is the incidence of nerve entrapment (defined as highly localised, sharp, stabbing or aching pain, exacerbated by particular movements and persisting beyond 5 weeks or occurring after a pain free interval) after one Pfannenstiel incision?

A. 1.7%

B. 3.7%

C. 5.7%

D. 7.7%

E. 9.7%

GTG 41 The Initial Management of Chronic Pelvic Pain

Nerve entrapment in scar tissue, fascia or a narrow foramen may result in pain and dysfunction in the distribution of that nerve.

The incidence of nerve entrapment (defined as highly localised, sharp, stabbing or aching pain, exacerbated by particular movements and persisting beyond 5 weeks or occurring after a pain free interval) after one Pfannenstiel incision is 3.7%.

250 A 22-year-old girl presents with lower abdominal pain, which is cyclical in nature.

Which modality is the only way to reliably diagnose peritoneal endometriosis?

A. Computerised Tomography Scan of the abdomen and pelvis

B. Laparoscopy

C. Magnetic Resonance Imaging of the abdomen and pelvis

D. Trans-abdominal ultrasound scan of the abdomen

E. Trans-vaginal ultrasound scan of the pelvis

GTG 41 The Initial Management of Chronic Pelvic Pain

In the past, diagnostic laparoscopy has been regarded as the 'gold standard' in the diagnosis of chronic pelvic pain. It may be considered as a second-line investigation if other therapeutic interventions fail.

Diagnostic laparoscopy may have a role in developing a woman's beliefs about her pain.

Diagnostic laparoscopy is the only test capable of reliably diagnosing peritoneal endometriosis and adhesions.

251 An 18-year-old girl with pelvic pain presents to the gynaecology outpatient clinic.

An ultrasound scan is arranged, which demonstrates a normal pelvis. Hormonal treatment is discussed with the girl.

How long should she persist with this therapy before contemplating a laparoscopy?

A. 1–3 months

B. 3–6 months

C. 6–9 months

D. 9–12 months

E. 1 year

GTG 41 The Initial Management of Chronic Pelvic Pain

Women with cyclical pain should be offered a therapeutic trial using hormonal treatment for a period of 3–6 months before having a diagnostic laparoscopy.

252 What proportion of the female adult population will complain of chronic pelvic pain?

   A. 1 in 2
   B. 1 in 4
   C. 1 in 6
   D. 1 in 10
   E. 1 in 20

GTG 41 The Initial Management of Chronic Pelvic Pain

Chronic pelvic pain is common, affecting perhaps one in six of the adult female population.

Much remains unclear about its aetiology, but chronic pelvic pain should be seen as a symptom with a number of contributory factors rather than as a diagnosis in itself. As with all chronic pain, it is important to consider psychological and social factors as well as physical causes of pain.

Many non-gynaecological conditions such as nerve entrapment or IBS may be relevant. Women often present because they seek an explanation for their pain.

253 A 19 year old has been seen in the gynaecology clinic with abdominal pain, which improves with defecation. It is associated with change in frequency of stool and change in form, for at least 3 days per month in the past 3 months.

What are the criteria used to define IBS?

   A. Amsterdam criteria
   B. Milan II criteria
   C. Rome III criteria
   D. Vienna II criteria
   E. Zurich criteria

GTG 41 The Initial Management of Chronic Pelvic Pain

APPENDIX 1: Rome III criteria for the diagnosis of IBS.

Continuous or recurrent abdominal pain or discomfort on at least 3 days a month in the past 3 months, with the onset at least 6 months previously, associated with at least two of the following: improvement with defecation, **onset** associated with a change in frequency of stool and onset associated with a change in the form of stool.

Symptoms such as abdominal bloating and the passage of mucus are commonly present and are suggestive of IBS. Extra intestinal symptoms such as lethargy, backache, urinary frequency and dyspareunia may also occur in association with IBS.

254 A 21 year old presents to the gynaecology outpatient clinic with pelvic pain. The general practitioner referral suggests possible endometriosis.

What is the estimated prevalence of endometriosis in women of reproductive age?

A. <1%

B. 2–10%

C. 10–20%

D. 25%

E. 50%

ESHRE guideline: Management of Women with Endometriosis

The exact prevalence of endometriosis is unknown but estimates range from 2 to 10% in women of reproductive age, to 50% in infertile women.

255 A 15-year-old girl is seen in the paediatric gynaecology clinic due to persistent vaginal discharge.

Examination reveals the following:

Partial removal of the clitoris and the prepuce is noted. The hymen is intact.

The possibility of female genital mutilation (FGM) is raised.

What type of FGM is this?

A. Type I

B. Type II

C. Type III

D. Type IV

E. It is not classed as FGM

GTG 53 Female Genital Mutilation and its Management

Partial or total removal of the clitoris and/or the prepuce (clitoridectomy).

Partial or total removal of the clitoris and the labia minora, with or without excision of the labia majora (excision).

Narrowing of the vaginal orifice with creation of a covering seal by cutting and appositioning the labia minora and/or the labia majora, with or without excision of the clitoris (infibulation).

All other harmful procedures to the female genitalia for nonmedical purposes, for example, pricking, piercing*, incising, scraping and cauterising.

*Piercing is part of this WHO classification but the legal status of this is unclear in the United Kingdom.

256 A 21 year old who complains of superficial dyspareunia is seen in the gynaecology clinic. She has just started her first ever sexual relationship.

On examination, the following features are noted:

Normal vulva and vagina. Clitoris is intact. A piercing is noted in the right labium minorum.

What type of FGM is this?

A. Type I
B. Type II
C. Type III
D. Type IV
E. It is not classed as FGM

GTG 53 Female Genital Mutilation and its Management

Partial or total removal of the clitoris and/or the prepuce (clitoridectomy).

Partial or total removal of the clitoris and the labia minora, with or without excision of the labia majora (excision).

Narrowing of the vaginal orifice with creation of a covering seal by cutting and appositioning the labia minora and/or the labia majora, with or without excision of the clitoris (infibulation).

All other harmful procedures to the female genitalia for non-medical purposes, e.g. pricking, piercing*, incising, scraping and cauterising.

*Piercing is part of this WHO classification but the legal status of this is unclear in the United Kingdom.

257 A 33-year-old woman is newly arrived in the United Kingdom from Africa and is complaining of dyspareunia.

How many women undergo FGM each year according to WHO estimates?

A. 500,000
B. 1 million
C. 2 million
D. 5 million
E. 10 million

GTG 53 Female Genital Mutilation and its Management

It is estimated by the WHO that 130 million women worldwide have undergone genital mutilation and that some two million women undergo some form of genital mutilation annually.

Traditionally, FGM is practised mainly in Africa but it is also found, to a lesser extent, in India and Indonesia. With increasing migration, obstetricians, gynaecologists and midwives in other parts of the world are encountering this practice and its complications (both acute and chronic), with increasing frequency. Within these countries, genital mutilation is not limited to any cultural or religious group.

258 A 24 year old has been seen in the antenatal clinic and is known to have undergone FGM. The lead midwife and health visitor are aware that any female offspring will be at risk of undergoing FGM. What is the estimated number of children in the United Kingdom that are considered to be at risk of this each year?

A. 500

B. 1000

C. 5000

D. 10,000

E. 20,000

GTG 53 Female Genital Mutilation and its Management

In countries in which FGM is illegal, families wanting the procedure for their young girls are likely to seek a traditional circumciser from their own community but some may approach health-care workers. To avoid detection, some girls may be taken abroad 'on holiday' and the procedure carried out there. There is a clear duty of child protection if a doctor is approached to perform a mutilating procedure or if it becomes known to them that a child is to be taken abroad for that purpose. It is estimated that 20,000 girls in the United Kingdom are at risk.

259 A 13 year old attends the Accident & Emergency department with bleeding, pain and urinary retention following a recent FGM. Which vaccine would you advise the patient to receive?

A. Hepatitis A

B. Hepatitis B

C. Hepatitis C

D. Tetanus toxoid

E. Varicella Zoster

GTG 53 Female Genital Mutilation and its Management

Females admitted acutely after FGM should be assessed quickly for signs of acute blood loss and sepsis, offered analgesia and tetanus toxoid vaccination if this had not previously been administered.

260 What is the most common cause of central precocious puberty (CPP) in girls?
   A. Craniopharyngioma
   B. Hydrocephalus
   C. Hypothalamic hamartoma
   D. Idiopathic
   E. McCune–Albright syndrome

TOG Article

Tirumuru SS, Arya P, Latthe P. Understanding precocious puberty in girls. The Obstetrician & Gynaecologist 2012;14:121–29.

The majority (74%) of girls have idiopathic CPP, but it can be secondary to an underlying disorder.

261 A 47-year-old Para 3 who has had three previous vaginal deliveries presents with a history of HMB that has not responded to medical treatment or the levonorgestrel-containing intrauterine system (LNG-IUS). The patient was offered endometrial ablation but declined.

On examination, the uterus is bulky, no masses palpable in the adnexa and the cervix descends to about 2 cm above the hymenal ring. An ultrasound confirms the physical examination findings. What is the most appropriate treatment option?
   A. A combination of endometrial resection and levonorgestrel releasing-IUS
   B. Laparoscopic vaginal assisted hysterectomy as it enables the surgeon to assess the pelvic organs
   C. Subtotal hysterectomy as it avoids possible bladder injury and has a lower incidence of sexual dysfunction
   D. Total abdominal hysterectomy as there is a lower risk of bladder injury than a vaginal hysterectomy
   E. Vaginal hysterectomy

NICE CG 44 Heavy Menstrual Bleeding

A vaginal hysterectomy has a lower risk of bladder injury than does abdominal hysterectomy. There is some descent of the uterus in a parous patient, therefore making the option of a vaginal hysterectomy a feasible option. A subtotal hysterectomy has a lower risk of bladder injury but does not have a lower incidence of sexual dysfunction. Laparoscopic vaginal hysterectomy might have been a useful option but an ultrasound scan ruled out the pelvic pathology and there is the added risk of laparoscopic surgery.

Taking into account the need for individual assessment, the route of hysterectomy should be considered in the following order: first line vaginal, second line abdominal.

262 An asymptomatic postmenopausal woman is diagnosed with a simple unilateral unilocular cyst with a diameter of 4.5 cm. Her serum CA125 is 10 iu/l.

What is the most appropriate first line of management?

A. Discharge to GP

B. Follow up with ultrasound in 4 months time

C. Laparoscopic Bilateral salpingo-oophorectomy

D. Laparoscopic Unilateral salpingo-oophorectomy

E. Total abdominal hysterectomy with Bilateral salpingo-oophorectomy

GTG 34 Ovarian Cysts in Postmenopausal Women

Simple, unilateral, unilocular ovarian cysts, less than 5 cm in diameter, have a low risk of malignancy. It is recommended that, in the presence of a normal serum CA125 levels, they be managed conservatively.

263 The prevalence of ovarian cysts in premenopausal woman is higher than that in postmenopausal women; 35% versus 17% respectively.

A premenopausal woman presents with an asymptomatic 4.5 cm simple cyst in the left ovary with a serum CA125 of 18 iu/l.

What would be the recommended management plan?

A. Aspiration of the cyst under ultrasound guidance

B. Aspiration of the cyst under direct laparoscopic view

C. Hysterectomy in addition to bilateral salpingo-oophorectomy

D. Laparoscopic left salpingo-oophorectomy

E. Reassure and manage conservatively

GTG 62 Management of Suspected Ovarian Masses in Premenopausal Women

The Society of Radiologists in Ultrasound published a consensus statement concluding that asymptomatic simple cysts 30–50 mm in diameter do not require follow-up, whereas cysts 50–70 mm require follow-up, and cysts more than 70 mm in diameter should be considered for either further imaging (MRI) or surgical intervention due to difficulties in examining the entire cyst adequately at the time of ultrasound.

264 A 40-year-old woman complains of burning and stinging in the vulva. There is no clinically identifiable neurological condition and there are no relevant visible findings.

What is the most likely clinical diagnosis?

A. Atrophic vaginitis

B. Herpes neuralgia

C. Immunobullous disorder

D. Lichen planus

E. Vulvodynia

TOG Article

Nagandla K, Sivalingam N. Vulvodynia: integrating current knowledge into clinical practice. The Obstetrician & Gynaecologist 2014;16:259–67.

The international Society for the study of Vulvo-vaginal disease (ISSVD) defines Vulvodynia as 'vulval discomfort that is described as burning, stinging or irritation in the absence of relevant visible findings or a specific signs of clinically identifiable neurological condition'.

265 A women diagnosed with localised unprovoked vulvodynia has had no relief from her symptoms despite practising good vulval care and using topical treatments which included lidocaine ointment and gabapentin.

What is the next line of management?

A. Anticonvulsant therapy

B. Laser ablation of Vulva

C. Modified vestibulectomy

D. Transcutaneous electrical nerve stimulation

E. Tricyclic antidepressant drugs

TOG Article
Nagandla K, Sivalingam N. Vulvodynia: integrating current knowledge into clinical practice. The Obstetrician & Gynaecologist 2014;16:259–67.

A prospective nonrandomised study demonstrated that women with unprovoked Vulvodynia who are prescribed TCAs had 47% reduction in their pain score.

266 Community-based surveys indicate that about one-fifth of women have significant vulval symptoms.
Symptoms and signs of vulval skin disorders are common and include pruritus, pain and changes in skin colour and texture.
What is the most common vulval disorder seen in a hospital setting?
A. Dermatitis
B. Lichen planus
C. Lichen sclerosus
D. Lichen simplex
E. Vulval Candidiasis

GTG 58 Management of Vulval Skin Disorders
Lichen sclerosus accounts for at least 25% of the women seen in dedicated vulval clinics, with estimates of incidence quoted as 1 in 300 to 1 in 1000 of all patients referred to dermatology departments.

267 Lichen sclerosus accounts for at least 25% of the women seen in dedicated vulval clinics, with estimates of incidence quoted as 1 in 300 to 1 in 1000 of all patients referred to dermatology departments.
What is the pathognomonic histologic feature of lichen sclerosus?
A. Acanthosis, hyperkeratosis and upper dermal fibrosis
B. Hyalisation of upper dermis
C. Plasma cells in a dense inflammatory infilterate
D. Squamous hyperplasia and a chronic perivascular inflammation
E. Thinning and effacement of the squamous epithelium with chronic upper dermal inflammation

Gynaecological and Obstetric Pathology for the MRCOG
Hyalization of upper dermis is a pathognomonic histologic feature of lichen sclerosus, which occurs in no other skin disease.

268 A 60-year-old woman presents with vulval itching with no relief with scratching.

On examination the skin appears fragile, with well demarcated white plaques. There is no involvement of the vagina or the oral mucosa.

What is the most likely diagnosis?

A. Lichen Planus

B. Lichen sclerosus

C. Lichen simplex chronicus

D. Vulval dermatitis

E. Vulval psoriasis

Gynaecological and Obstetric Pathology for the MRCOG

Lichen sclerosus almost never involves the vagina and the oral mucosa.

269 A woman with biopsy-proven lichen sclerosus is not responding to topical ultra-potent steroids.

What is the second line of treatment?

A. CO_2 Laser vaporisation

B. Local surgical excision

C. Topical emollient

D. Topical imiquimod cream

E. Topical Tacrolimus

GTG 58 Management of Vulval Skin Disorders

Tacrolimus is a calcineurin inhibitor. The mode of action differs from that of corticosteroids, mainly reducing inflammation by suppressing T-lymphocyte responses. Tacrolimus has been shown to be effective at controlling a number of vulval dermatoses including lichen sclerosus and lichen planus.

270 A 25-year-old smoker is diagnosed to have mild dyskariosis in her index smear at the GP surgery. The smear is HPV negative.

What is the ideal management?

A. Reassure and discharge for repeat smear in 3 years

B. Referral to colposcopy for review

C. Repeat smear in 12 months and if still has mild dyskariosis refer for colposcopy

D. Repeat smear in 3 months and if still has mild dyskariosis refer for colposcopy

E. Repeat smear in 6 months and if still has mild dyskariosis refer for colposcopy

NHS Cervical Screening Programme

Women who have borderline/mild dyskariosis on smear but are HPV negative can be reassured and discharged to routine smear.

271 A 40-year-old woman attends for a consultation in primary care complaining of HMB. She is otherwise fit and well and examination is unremarkable.

What investigation should be undertaken?

A. Coagulation screen

B. Endometrial biopsy

C. Full blood count

D. Pelvic ultrasound scan

E. Serum ferritin

NICE CG 44 Heavy Menstrual Bleeding

A full blood count test should be carried out on all women with HMB. This should be done in parallel with any HMB treatment offered.

Testing for coagulation disorders (e.g., von Willebrand's disease) should be considered in women who have had HMB since menarche and have personal or family history suggesting a coagulation disorder.

A serum ferritin test should not routinely be carried out on women with HMB.

Imaging should be performed in the following circumstances:

The uterus is palpable abdominally

Vaginal examination reveals a pelvic mass of uncertain origin

Pharmaceutical treatment fails

Ultrasound is the first-line diagnostic tool.

272 Following referral to secondary care for HMB, a 38-year old woman undergoes pelvic examination, which confirms that the uterus is palpable abdominally.

What is the first line diagnostic test to identify structural abnormalities in this situation?

A. CT scan

B. Hysteroscopy

C. MRI scan

D. Pelvic ultrasound scan

E. Saline infusion sonography

NICE CG 44 Heavy Menstrual Bleeding

Imaging should be performed in the following circumstances:

The uterus is palpable abdominally

Vaginal examination reveals a pelvic mass of uncertain origin

Pharmaceutical treatment fails

Ultrasound is the first-line diagnostic tool for identifying structural abnormalities

Saline infusion sonography should not be used as a first-line diagnostic tool

Magnetic resonance imaging (MRI) should not be considered as a first-line diagnostic tool.

273 A 39-year-old woman presents to the gynaecology clinic with HMB and dysmenorrhoea. She is otherwise fit and well.

Pelvic examination is unremarkable.

She is not keen on hormonal methods of treatment.

What treatment would you initially recommend?

A. Danazol

B. Etamsylate

C. Mefenemic acid

D. Norethisterone

E. Tranexamic acid

NICE CG 44 Heavy Menstrual Bleeding

When HMB coexists with dysmenorrhoea, NSAIDs should be preferred to tranexamic acid.

Danazol should not be used routinely for the treatment of HMB.

Etamsylate should not be used for the treatment of HMB.

274 A 38-year-old woman is seen in the gynaecology clinic. She presented with HMB.

History and examination are unremarkable and she is commenced on tranexamic acid, to be taken during menstruation only.

Should this treatment ultimately prove to be ineffective, for how many cycles should she have tried it to come to this conclusion?

A. 3 cycles

B. 6 cycles

C. 9 cycles

D. 12 cycles

E. 18 cycles

NICE CG 44 Heavy Menstrual bleeding

Use of NSAIDs and/or tranexamic acid should be stopped if it does not improve symptoms within three menstrual cycles.

275 During investigation for HMB, a 42-year-old woman is found to have a 3 cm submucus fibroid.

She is otherwise fit and well. Her husband has had a vasectomy.
She does not wish to try pharmaceutical treatments.
What would you recommend?

A. Hysteroscopic resection of fibroid and endometrium
B. Novasure endometrial ablation
C. Open myomectomy
D. Total abdominal hysterectomy
E. Uterine artery embolisation

NICE CG 44 Heavy Menstrual Bleeding

In women with HMB alone, with uterus no bigger than a 10-week pregnancy, endometrial ablation should be considered in preference to hysterectomy.

First-generation ablation techniques (e.g., rollerball endometrial ablation [REA] and transcervical resection of the endometrium [TCRE]) are appropriate if hysteroscopic myomectomy is to be included in the procedure.

UAE, myomectomy or hysterectomy should be considered in cases of HMB where large fibroids (greater than 3 cm in diameter) are present and bleeding is having a severe impact on a woman's quality of life.

276 A 55-year-old woman attends the general practitioner surgery with abdominal distension, low abdominal pain and urinary urgency.

Abdominal examination is unremarkable and urine dipstick is negative.
What investigation should be performed?

A. CT scan urinary tract
B. Full blood count
C. No investigation – reassure and discharge
D. Pelvic ultrasound scan
E. Serum CA125

NICE CG 122 Ovarian Cancer

Carry out tests in primary care if a woman (especially if 50 or over) reports having any of the following symptoms on a persistent or frequent basis – particularly more than 12 times per month:

> persistent abdominal distension (women often refer to this as 'bloating')
> feeling full (early satiety) and/or loss of appetite
> pelvic or abdominal pain
> increased urinary urgency and/or frequency.
> Measure serum CA125 in primary care in women with symptoms that suggest ovarian cancer.

277 What screening test should be offered to all sexually active women who present to the gynaecology clinic with chronic pelvic pain?

A. Endocervical swabs for Chlamydia and Gonorrhoea

B. Magnetic resonance imaging

C. Serum CA125

D. Serum C-reactive protein

E. Transvaginal ultrasound

GTG 41 Chronic Pelvic Pain

All sexually active women with chronic pelvic pain should be offered screening for sexually transmitted infections (STIs).

278 After a year of 4-monthly follow-up, a healthy 75-year-old woman with a 5 cm simple unilocular ovarian cyst and a normal serum CA-125 level decides that she would prefer to have surgical treatment.

What treatment would you recommend?

A. Aspiration of the cyst

B. Laparoscopic bilateral oophorectomy

C. Laparoscopic ovarian cystectomy

D. Laparoscopic unilateral oophorectomy

E. Total abdominal hysterectomy and bilateral salpingo-oophorectomy

GTG 34 Ovarian Cysts in Postmenopausal Women

Aspiration is not recommended for the management of ovarian cysts in postmenopausal women.

It is recommended that laparoscopic management of ovarian cysts in postmenopausal women should involve oophorectomy (usually bilateral) rather than cystectomy.

279 Following a diagnosis of anogenital lichen sclerosus, a 70-year-old woman returns to clinic as topical potent steroids have not been effective in controlling her symptoms.

The recommended second-line treatment is Tacrolimus.

Which cell type of the immune system has its response suppressed by this drug?

A. B lymphocytes

B. Macrophages

C. Natural killer cells

D. Plasma cells

E. T lymphocytes

GTG 58 The Management of Vulval Skin Disorders

Tacrolimus and pimicrolimus belong to the class of immunosuppressant drugs known as calcineurin inhibitors. Their mode of action differs from that of corticosteroids, in mainly reducing inflammation by suppressing T-lymphocyte responses.

280 Which progestagen has been shown to be effective in cases of PMS?

A. Desogestrel

B. Drospirenone

C. Levonorgestrel

D. Medroxyprogesterone acetate

E. Norethisterone

GTG 48 Management of Premenstrual Syndrome

Progestogen in the second-generation pills (i.e., levonorgestrel or norethisterone) regenerate PMS-type symptoms. A new combined contraceptive pill (Yasmin®, Schering Health) contains an antimineralocorticoid and antiandrogenic progestogen, drospirenone. Initial studies suggest that this is beneficial. There are data from observational and small randomised trials supporting its efficacy.

Module 14

Subfertility

281 A 28-year-old amenorrhoeic woman who wishes to become pregnant attends the fertility clinic complaining of galactorrhoea and mild visual disturbance. Her serum prolactin level was found to be elevated.

An MRI scan of the head is performed, which showed the presence of a macroprolactinoma, but without supracellar extension.

What is the most appropriate first line management?

A. Bromocriptine

B. Cabergoline

C. Quinagolide

D. Radiotherapy

E. Trans-sphenoidal surgical excision of the prolactinoma

TOG Article

Hamoda H, Khalaf Y, Carroll P. Hyperprolactinaemia and female reproductive function: what does the evidence say? The Obstetrician & Gynaecologist 2012;14:81–86.

Treatment of hyperprolactinemia in women who wish to have a pregnancy is dependent on the size of the prolactinoma and its clinical presentation. Medical treatment is preferred to surgery where possible and will generally provide optimal control in most cases with microprolactinomas or macroprolactinomas with no supracellar extension. Because of its better established safety profile, bromocriptine is generally the first line of treatment.

282 In the female, which cell type secretes Anti-Mullerian hormone?

A. Granulosa cells

B. Leydig cells

C. Primary oocytes

D. Secondary Oocytes

E. Sertoli cells

Part 2 MRCOG: Single Best Answer Questions, First Edition.
Andrew Sizer, Chandrika Balachandar, Nibedan Biswas, Richard Foon, Anthony Griffiths, Sheena Hodgett, Banchhita Sahu and Martyn Underwood.
© 2016 John Wiley & Sons, Ltd. Published 2016 by John Wiley & Sons, Ltd.

TOG Article

Bhide P, Shah A, Gudi A, Homburg R. The role of anti-mullerian hormone as a predictor of ovarian function. The Obstetrician & Gynaecologist 2012;14:161–166.

AMH is a glycoprotein belonging to the transforming growth factor β family. In the male fetus it is expressed in the Sertoli cells of the testes, which leads to Mullerian regression. In the female fetus it is expressed by the granulosa cells of the ovary from as early as 36 weeks of gestation and production continues until menopause.

283 A woman with tubal disease is advised to have IVF treatment to maximise her chances of pregnancy. On reading the information leaflet, she is very concerned about the risks of ovarian hyperstimulation syndrome.

What is the chance of developing severe ovarian hyperstimulation syndrome (OHSS) and requiring hospitalisation in women undergoing controlled ovarian hyperstimulation?

A. 0.1–0.2 %
B. 1–3%
C. 8–10%
D. 15–20%
E. 30–40%

TOG Article

Bhide P, Shah A, Gudi A, Homburg R. The role of anti-Mullerian hormone as a predictor of ovarian function. The Obstetrician & Gynaecologist 2012;14:161–166.

Among the women undergoing controlled ovarian hyperstimulation for IVF, 15–20% have mild to moderate OHSS and 1–3% have severe OHSS and require hospitalisation.

284 What is the predominant cause of anovulatory infertility?
A. Hyperprolactinemia
B. Hypogonadotrophic hypogonadism
C. Obesity
D. Polycystic ovary syndrome
E. Premature ovarian failure

TOG Article

Gorthi S, Balen AH, Tang T. Current issues in ovulation induction. The Obstetrician & Gynaecologist 2012;14:188–196.

Polycystic ovary syndrome (PCOS; group II) is the predominant cause of anovulatory infertility, accounting for >80–90% of all cases.

285 What is the first-line pharmacological treatment for anovulatory polycystic ovary syndrome?
A. Anastrozole
B. Clomifene
C. Letrozole
D. Recombinant FSH
E. Tamoxifen

TOG Article

Gorthi S, Balen AH, Tang T. Current issues in ovulation induction. The Obstetrician & Gynaecologist 2012;14:188–196.

The Thessaloniki ESHRE/ASRM-Sponsored PCOS Consensus Workshop Group recommends that clomifene is still used as the first-line treatment for an ovulatory PCOS.

286 A 32-year-old woman presents to the gynaecology clinic with galactorrhoea and secondary amenorrhoea. A serum prolactin level is measured and found to be elevated.
What is the main mechanism by which hyperprolactinemia causes secondary amenorrhoea?
A. Disruption of granulosa cell development
B. Induction of atrophic changes in the endometrium
C. Inhibition of follicle stimulating hormone (FSH) pulsatility
D. Inhibition of Luteinising hormone (LH) pulsatility
E. Inhibition of meiosis in the developing oocyte

TOG Article

Hamoda H, Khalaf Y, Carroll P. Hyperprolactinaemia and female reproductive function: what does the evidence say? The Obstetrician & Gynaecologist 2012;14:81–86.

In 1974, McNatty showed that high levels of prolactin result in anovulation, secondary to inhibition of luteinising hormone pulsatility.

287 Following an IVF treatment cycle where 15 oocytes were collected, a patient presents to the clinic with abdominal pain, nausea and vomiting.

An ultrasound scan is performed, which shows the ovaries to be enlarged with a mean diameter of 10 cm. There is a small amount of ascites.

What is the diagnosis?

A. Critical OHSS

B. Mild OHSS

C. Moderate OHSS

D. Normal findings post oocyte-retrieval

E. Severe OHSS

GTG 5 The Management of Ovarian Hyperstimulation Syndrome

Table 1.	Classification of severity of OHSS
Grade	**Symptoms**
Mild OHSS	Abdominal bloating
	Mild abdominal pain
	Ovarian size usually <8 cm*
Moderate OHSS	Moderate abdominal pain
	Nausea ± vomiting
	Ultrasound evidence of ascites
	Ovarian size usually 8–12 cm*
Severe OHSS	Clinical ascites (occasionally hydrothorax)
	Oliguria
	Haemoconcentration haematocrit >45%
	Hypoproteinaemia
	Ovarian size usually >12 cm*
Critical OHSS	Tense ascites or large hydrothorax
	Haematocrit >55%
	White cell count >25 000/ml
	Oligo/anuria
	Thromboembolism
	Acute respiratory distress syndrome

288 What type of electrolyte disturbance is often seen in association with severe cases of OHSS?

A. Hypercalcaemia

B. Hyperkalaemia

C. Hypernatraemia

D. Hypokalaemia

E. Hyponatraemia

GTG 5 The Management of Ovarian Hyperstimulation Syndrome

Hyponatraemia, observed in 56% cases of severe OHSS, may be dilutional as a result of antidiurectic hormone hypersecretion.

289 A woman with a severe cases of OHSS initially presented with tense ascites, oliguria and a haematocrit of 46%.

She was treated with appropriate fluid replacement and the haematocrit is now in the normal range.

However, she remains markedly oliguric.

What is the appropriate management?

A. Bendroflumethazide orally

B. Furosemide IV

C. Haemodialysis

D. Ongoing intravenous fluids at a rate of 5–6 l/24 hours

E. Paracentesis

GTG 5 The Management of Ovarian Hyperstimulation Syndrome

Paracentesis should be considered in women who are distressed due to abdominal distension or in whom oliguria persists despite adequate volume replacement.

Diuretics should not be used in women with oliguria secondary to a reduced blood volume and decreased renal perfusion, as they may worsen intravascular dehydration. Where oliguria persists despite adequate rehydration (preferably judged by invasive haemodynamic monitoring), rarely there may be a role for the judicious use of diuretics with senior multidisciplinary involvement and usually after paracentesis.

290 What is the recommended test for the biochemical detection of hyperandrogenism?

A. 17-hydroxy progesterone

B. Free androgen index

C. Free testosterone

D. Sex-hormone binding globulin

E. Total testosterone

GTG 33 Long-Term Consequences of Polycystic Ovary Syndrome

Although free and total testosterone is used in the diagnosis of PCOS, the recommended baseline biochemical test for hyperandrogenism is free androgen index (total amount of testosterone divided by the quantity of sex hormone binding globulin [SHBG] × 100).

291 What proportion of women with polycystic ovarian syndrome are overweight/obese?

A. 10–20%

B. 40–50%

C. 60–70%

D. 80–85%

E. 95–100%

SiP 13 Metformin Therapy for the Management of Infertility in Women with Polycystic Ovary Syndrome

The consensus definition of PCOS recognises obesity as an association and not as a diagnostic criterion as only 40–50% of women with PCOS are overweight.

292 What is the mechanism of action of Metformin?

A. Enhances insulin sensitivity at the cellular level

B. Increases renal glucose reabsorption

C. Inhibits insulin release

D. Promotes hepatic glycogenolysis

E. Promotes hepatic gluconeogenesis

SiP 13 Metformin Therapy for the Management of Infertility in Women with Polycystic Ovary Syndrome

Metformin inhibits the production of hepatic glucose, enhances insulin sensitivity at the cellular level and also appears to have direct effects on ovarian function.

293 What is the estimated prevalence of endometriosis in infertile women?

A. 10%

B. 20%

C. 30%

D. 40%

E. 50%

ESHRE Guideline: Management of Women with Endometriosis

The exact prevalence of endometriosis is unknown but estimates range from 2% to 10% in women of reproductive age, to 50% of infertile women.

294 During fertility investigations, a woman is found to be susceptible to Rubella and is offered vaccination.

How long should she use contraception before trying to conceive again?

A. 1 month

B. 3 months

C. 6 months

D. 12 months

E. Can try and conceive immediately

NICE CG156 Fertility

Women who are concerned about their fertility should be offered testing for their rubella status so that those who are susceptible to rubella can be offered vaccination. Women who are susceptible to rubella should be offered vaccination and advised not to become pregnant for at least 1 month following vaccination.

295 Following fertility investigations, a man is found to have idiopathic oligozoospermia.

He enquires if there is any treatment he can take to improve his sperm count.

What would you recommend?

A. Androstenedione

B. Clomiphene citrate

C. Letrozole

D. No treatment is of proven benefit

E. Recombinant FSH

NICE CG156 Fertility

Men with idiopathic semen abnormalities should not be offered antioestrogens, gonadotrophins, androgens, bromocriptine or kinin-enhancing drugs because they have not been shown to be effective.

296 Following a full set of investigations in the fertility clinic, a couple are diagnosed as having unexplained infertility since all the tests have been reported as normal.

The couple have been trying to conceive for 3 years.

What treatment would be recommended?

A. Conservative management

B. Ovulation induction with Clomiphene citrate

C. Ovulation induction with Letrozole

D. Intracytoplasmic sperm injection (ICSI)

E. In vitro fertilisation (IVF)

NICE CG 156 Fertility

Offer IVF treatment to women with unexplained infertility who have not conceived after 2 years (this can include up to 1 year before their fertility investigations) of regular unprotected sexual intercourse.

Do not offer oral ovarian stimulation agents (such as clomifene citrate, anastrozole or letrozole) to women with unexplained infertility.

297 Prior to a frozen embryo transfer, a woman takes a course of oestradiol valerate to induce endometrial proliferation.

She attends for an ultrasound scan after 10 days to measure the endometrial thickness.

What endometrial thickness should have been achieved in order for the embryo transfer to proceed?

A. 1 mm
B. 2 mm
C. 3 mm
D. 4 mm
E. 5 mm

NICE CG 156 Fertility

Replacement of embryos into a uterine cavity with an endometrium of less than 5 mm thickness is unlikely to result in a pregnancy and is therefore not recommended.

298 Which form of contraception is most strongly associated with a delay in return of fertility?

A. Copper-containing intrauterine device
B. Depo medroxyprogesterone acetate
C. Etonorgestrel-containing subdermal implant
D. Levonorgestrel containing intrauterine system
E. Progestogen-only pill

NICE CG 30 Long-Acting Reversible Contraception

There could be a delay of up to 1 year in the return of fertility after stopping the use of injectable contraceptives.

299 Fertility declines with age.
What percentage of women aged 35 will take longer than a year to conceive with regular intercourse?
A. 5%
B. 15%
C. 30%
D. 45%
E. 60%

TOG Article

Utting D, Bewley S. Family planning and age-related reproductive risk. The Obstetrician & Gynaecologist 2011;13:35–41.

At the age of 25, only 5% of women take longer than a year to conceive with regular intercourse, with the percentage rising to 30 in those aged 35.

300 According to the current WHO criteria, what is the reference limit for the total number of spermatozoa in an ejaculate?
A. 4×10^6
B. 15×10^6
C. 32×10^6
D. 39×10^6
E. 58×10^6

TOG Article

Karavolos S, Stewart J, Evbuomwan I, McEleny K, Aird I. Assessment of the infertile male. The Obstetrician & Gynaecologist 2013;15:1–9.

Table 1. World Health Organization reference limits and 95% confidence intervals for semen parameters[48]

Parameter	Reference limit	95% confidence interval
Semen volume (ml)	1.5	1.4–1.7
Sperm concentration (10^6/ml)	15.0	12–16
Total number (10^6/ejaculate)	39.0	33–46
Total motility (PR+NP, %)	40.0	38–42
Progressive motility (PR, %)	32.0	31–34
Normal forms (%)	4.0	3.0–4.0
Vitality (%)	58.0	55–63

NP = non-progressive motility; PR = progressive motility

Module 15

Sexual and Reproductive Health

301 In the United Kingdom, which synthetic oestrogen is contained in most combined oral contraceptive (COC) pills?
A. Cyproterone acetate
B. Drospirenone
C. Ethinylestradiol
D. Oestradiol valerate
E. Mestranol

FSRH Statement Venous Thromboembolism (VTE) and Hormonal Contraception

In the United Kingdom, the majority of combined hormonal contraceptives contains the synthetic oestrogen, ethinylestradiol. A COC product containing mestranol is also available, with 50 µg of mestranol roughly equating to 35 µg of ethinylestradiol.

More recently, COC products have been introduced into the market, which contain the naturally occurring human hormone, estradiol, either as estradiol valerate or as estradiol hemihydrate.

302 What is the primary mode of action of the progestogen-only injectable method of contraception (Depo Provera)?
A. Endometrial atrophy
B. Inhibition of ovulation
C. Prevention of fertilisation
D. Prevention of implantation
E. Thickening of cervical mucus

NICE CG 30 Long-Acting Reversible Contraception

Progestogen-only injectable contraceptives act primarily by preventing ovulation.

303 What is the most efficacious form of long-acting reversible contraception?

  A. COC pill
  B. Copper intrauterine device
  C. Depo medroxyprogesterone acetate
  D. Etonorgestrel-containing subdermal implant
  E. Levonorgestrel-containing intrauterine system

NICE CG 30 Long-Acting Reversible Contraception

	Copper IUD	IUS	Progestogen-only injection	Implant
How it works	By preventing fertilisation and inhibiting implantation	Mainly by preventing implantation; sometimes by preventing fertilisation	Primarily by preventing ovulation	Primarily by preventing ovulation
Duration of use	5–10 years for IUDs with 380 mm² copper, depending on type Until contraception no longer needed if woman 40 years or more at time of insertion[H]	5 years Until contraception no longer needed if woman 45 years or more at time of insertion and does not have periods with IUS in place[H]	Repeat injections needed every 12 weeks (DPMA) or 8 weeks (NET-EN)[H]	3 years
Failure rate	Fewer than 2 in 100 women over 5 years, for IUDs with at least 380 mm² copper Expulsion occurs in fewer than 1 in 20 women in 5 years	Fewer than 1 in 100 women over 5 years Expulsion occurs in fewer than 1 in 20 women in 5 years	Fewer than 0.4 in 100 over 2 years; pregnancy rates lower for DPMA than NET-EN	Fewer than 1 pregnancy in 1000 implants fitted over 3 years

304 Which form of progestogen-only contraception is most strongly associated with loss of bone mineral density?

  A. Depo medroxyprogesterone acetate
  B. Depo norethisterone enantate
  C. Etonorgestrel-containing subdermal implant
  D. Levonorgestrel-containing intrauterine system
  E. Progestogen-only pill

NICE CG 30 Long-Acting Reversible Contraception

DMPA use is associated with a small loss of bone mineral density, which is largely recovered when DMPA is discontinued.

305 Which form of long-acting reversible contraception is least suitable for use in adolescents?

A. COC pill

B. Copper intrauterine device

C. Depo medroxyprogesterone acetate

D. Etonorgestrel-containing subdermal implant

E. Levonorgestrel-containing intrauterine system

NICE CG 30 Long-Acting Reversible Contraception

Choices for adolescents:

IUD, IUS, implants: no specific restrictions to use.

DMPA: care needed; only use if other methods are unacceptable or are not suitable.

306 Which two drugs are the only selective progesterone receptor modulators (SPRMs) licensed for use in the United Kingdom?

A. Medroxyprogesterone acetate and Ulipristal acetate

B. Mifepristone and Misoprostol

C. Mifepristone and Tibolone

D. Mifepristone and Ulipristal acetate

E. Tibolone and Drospirenone

TOG Article

Murdoch M, Roberts M. Selective progesterone receptor modulators and their use within gynaecology. The Obstetrician & Gynaecologist, 2014;16:46–50.

Mifepristone and ulipristal acetate are the only SPRMs currently licensed for use in the United Kingdom; however, other SPRMs have been or are currently being developed and are undergoing trial.

307 What is the background rate of venous thromboembolism (VTE) in women of reproductive age?

A. 10/100,000/year

B. 20/100,000/year

C. 50/100,000/year

D. 100/100,000/year

E. 200/100,000/year

Faculty of Sexual and Reproductive Healthcare Statement
Venous Thromboembolism (VTE) and Hormonal Contraception
The true background incidence of VTE in women of reproductive age is difficult to quantify but recently published figures suggest that it is in the range of 2 per 10,000 women in 1 year.

308 A woman switches from a COC pill containing ethinyloestradiol and levonorgestrel to a different pill containing ethinyloestradiol and desogestrel. The dose of ethinyloestradiol is the same in both preparations.
Approximately, by how many times will she have increased her risk of VTE?
A. 2
B. 5
C. 10
D. 15
E. 20

Faculty of Sexual and Reproductive Healthcare Statement
Venous Thromboembolism (VTE) and Hormonal Contraception

Risk of VTE per 10,000 healthy women over 1 year	
Non contraceptive users and not pregnant	2
CHC containing ethinylestradiol plus levonorgestrel, norgestimate or norethisterone	5–7
CHC containing etonogestrel (ring) or norelgestromin (patch)	6–12
CHC containing ethinylestradiol plus gestodene, desogestrel or drospirenone	9–12

309 What is the primary mode of action by which the COC pill exerts its contraceptive effect?
A. Endometrial atrophy
B. Inhibition of ovulation
C. Sperm immobilisation
D. Suppression of meiosis
E. Thickening of cervical mucus

TOG Article

Carey MS, Allen RH. Non-contraceptive uses and benefits of combined oral contraception. The Obstetrician & Gynaecologist 2012;14:223–8.

COCs consist of an oestrogen in combination with a progestogen and work primarily by inhibiting ovulation.

310 What percentage of women with gonorrohea are coinfected with chlamydia?

    A. 10%
    B. 20%
    C. 30%
    D. 40%
    E. 50%

TOG Article

Allstaff S, Wilson J. The management of sexually transmitted infections in pregnancy. TOG 2012;14;25–32

Almost 40% of women with gonorrohea are coinfected with chlamydia. Therapeutic regimens should include chlamydia treatment due to the high rate of coinfection.

311 Gonorrohea infection in pregnancy increases the risk of preterm rupture of membranes, preterm birth and low birth weight.

    What percentage of exposed babies would develop Ophthalmia neonatorum?

    A. 50%
    B. 60%
    C. 70%
    D. 80%
    E. 90%

TOG Article

Allstaff S, Wilson J. The management of sexually transmitted infections in pregnancy. TOG 2012;14;25–32

Gonorrohea testing should be performed on women with lower genital tract symptoms, intrapartum or postpartum fever and mothers of infants with ophthalmia neonatorum. There is an increased rate of pharyngeal infection in pregnancy. Almost 40% of women are coinfected with chlamydia. Treatment regimen should include chlamydia treatment due to high rate of coinfection. Ophthalmia neonatorum occurs in up to 50% of exposed babies.

Treatment efficacy is not reduced in pregnancy. Amoxicillin with probenecid, spectinomycin, ceftriaxone and cefixime are equally effective, but because of emerging high levels of resistance, penicillins are not recommended.

312 Trichomonas vaginalis infection in pregnancy is associated with preterm birth and low birth weight.
What percentage of infected women are asymptomatic?
A. 10–50%
B. 50–60%
C. 60–70%
D. 70–80%
E. 80–90%

TOG Article
Allstaff S, Wilson J. The management of sexually transmitted infections in pregnancy. TOG 2012;14;25–32

Trichomonal vaginalis is associated with preterm birth and low birth weight.

10–50% of women infected are asymptomatic. Most common nonviral STI worldwide. Nitroimidazoles are the most effective treatment for Trichomonal vaginalis. There are insufficient safety data for tinidazole in pregnancy and its use cannot be recommended. A test of cure is recommended if symptoms fail to resolve or if symptoms recur.

313 Vertical transmission of human papilloma virus (HPV) can cause genital and laryngeal warts and recurrent respiratory papillomatosis in infants.
What is the risk of vertical transmission?
A. 1 in 1000 cases
B. 1 in 500 cases
C. 1 in 150 cases
D. 1 in 80 cases
E. 1 in 50 cases

TOG Article
Allstaff S, Wilson J. The management of sexually transmitted infections in pregnancy. TOG 2012;14;25–32.

Vertical transmission of HPV occurs in up to 1 in 80 cases and can cause genital and laryngeal warts in infants. Treatment of anogenital warts in pregnancy does not reduce the risk of vertical transmission.

314 Most cases of syphilis in pregnancy are detected through antenatal screening. The management should involve a multidisciplinary team of obstetricians, genitourinary physicians and neonatologists. Penicillin is the treatment of choice.

What percentage of cases develop the Jarisch–Herxheimer reaction during treatment of syphilis in pregnancy?

A. 5%

B. 25%

C. 45%

D. 65%

E. 85%

TOG Article

Allstaff S, Wilson J. The management of sexually transmitted infections in pregnancy. TOG 2012;14;25–32.

The Jarisch–Herxheimer reaction can complicate up to 45% of syphilis treatments in pregnancy. Management of the Jarisch–Herxheimer reaction should be supportive and should include antipyretics, but oral corticosteroids are not indicated.

315 Vasectomy failure rate is quoted as approximately 1 in 2000 (0.05%) after clearance has been given.

By how many months postprocedure should the vasectomy be considered a failure if motile sperm are still observed in a fresh semen sample?

A. 3 months

B. 4 months

C. 5 months

D. 6 months

E. 7 months

FSRH Clinical Guidance Male and Female Sterilisation

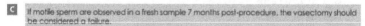

C If motile sperm are observed in a fresh sample 7 months post-procedure, the vasectomy should be considered a failure.

316 Ulipristal acetate (UPA) may itself reduce the efficacy of other hormonal contraception.

When emergency contraception is administered because of a missed combined oral contraceptive pill (CHC) the CHC should be continued.

For how many days should additional contraception be advised?

A. 0 days
B. 7 days
C. 14 days
D. 21 days
E. 28 days

FSRH Statement on Drug Interactions between Hormonal Contraception and Ulipristal Products: ellaOne® and Esmya®

Table 3 Faculty of Sexual & Reproductive Healthcare recommendations on additional contraception after emergency contraception in women using hormonal contraception

EC Options	Additional contraceptive precautions (condom or avoidance of sex)
Cu-IUD	No additional contraception required
LNG	7 days (2 for POP, 9 for Qlaira)
UPA	14 days (9 for POP, 16 for Qlaira)

317 Besides providing reliable contraception, COC offers a variety of noncontraceptive health benefits.
What percentage of women of reproductive age use COCs for contraception in the United Kingdom?
A. 7%
B. 17%
C. 27%
D. 37%
E. 47%

TOG Article

Carey MS, Allen RH. Non-contraceptive uses and benefits of combined oral contraception. The Obstetrician & Gynaecologist 2012;14:223–8.

In the United Kingdom, approximately 27% of women aged 16–49 years report using COCs for contraception.

318 Reproductive coercion is defined as the attempt by men to control their female partners' pregnancies and pregnancy outcomes.
What is the reported percentage of incidence of birth control sabotage by male partners?
A. 25%
B. 35%
C. 45%
D. 55%
E. 65%

TOG Article

Gottlieb AS. Domestic violence: a clinical guide for women's health care providers. The Obstetrician & Gynaecologist 2012;14:197–202.

As the largest assessment to date of reproductive coercion in the United States, Miller's research corroborates earlier studies, describing the lengths to which male partners will go to assert power over reproduction, such as poking holes in condoms, pulling out NuvaRings and flushing oral contraceptive pills down the toilet. The findings also support the association between domestic violence and unintended pregnancy demonstrated previously and potentially explain the relationship between these two phenomena. In Miller's study, approximately 35% of domestic violence victims reported birth control sabotage or forced pregnancy by their partners, with reproductive coercion in the setting of a partner abuse history doubling the risk of unintended pregnancy.

319 More and more women are leaving childbearing to a later age. What is the most common reason given by women for making this choice?

 A. Availability of reliable contraceptives
 B. Career concerns
 C. Financial reasons
 D. Finding a suitable partner
 E. Other causes

TOG Article

Utting D, Bewley S. Family planning and age-related reproductive risk. The Obstetrician & Gynaecologist 2011;13:35–41.

The mean age of childbearing was 23 years in 1968, 26.7 in 1978 and 29.3 in 2008. Women aged 30–34 have nearly doubled their fecundity in the last three decades, numerically overtaking women in the 25–29 age group for the first time in 2004. An ICM poll in 2006 cited numerous reasons given by women for later childbearing, the most common being career concerns (63%), financial reasons (53%) and finding a suitable partner (53%).

320 As a post coital contraception, the primary mechanism of action of Ulipristal acetate is inhibition of ovulation.

What is the conception rate when Ulipristal acetate is taken within 120 hours of unprotected sexual intercourse?

A. 1.3%

B. 2.3%

C. 3.3%

D. 4.3%

E. 5.3%

TOG Article

Bhathena RK, Guillebaud J. Postcoital contraception. The Obstetrician & Gynaecologist 2011;13:29–34.

The conception rates in women who were given emergency contraception 0–120 hours after unprotected intercourse were 1.3% for ulipristal acetate and 2.2% for levonorgestrel.

Module 16

Early Pregnancy Problems

321 A woman attends her first ultrasound scan in pregnancy. What is the maximum crown rump length (CRL) that is accurate for dating before you measure gestational age by head circumference (HC)
  A. 14 mm
  B. 24 mm
  C. 44 mm
  D. 84 mm
  E. 94 mm

NICE CG 62 Antenatal Care

Accurate dating is important and women should be offered an ultrasound scan between 10 weeks and 0 days to 13 weeks and 6 days.

CRL measurement should be used to determine gestational age. If the CRL is above 84 mm, the gestational age should be estimated using HC.

322 At what gestational age is chorionic villus sampling (CVS) usually performed?
  A. $8-10^{+0}$ gestation
  B. $8-13^{+6}$ gestation
  C. $10-11^{+0}$ gestation
  D. $11-13^{+6}$ gestation
  E. $12-14^{+6}$ gestation

GTG 8 Amniocentesis and Chorionic Villus Sampling

Chorionic villi sampling (CVS) is usually offered between 11+ 0 and 13 + 6 weeks of gestation. It can involve aspiration or biopsy of the placenta villi. The process of extraction can be performed transcervically

---

Part 2 MRCOG: Single Best Answer Questions, First Edition.
Andrew Sizer, Chandrika Balachandar, Nibedan Biswas, Richard Foon, Anthony Griffiths, Sheena Hodgett, Banchhita Sahu and Martyn Underwood.

or transabdominally. It is a common method of invasive fetal testing in the United Kingdom.

323 A woman is currently being treated for acne with oral retinoids and finds herself pregnant in the first trimester. What is her chance of miscarrying?

A. 5%

B. 10–15%

C. 20–40%

D. 30–50%

E. 80–90%

TOG Article

Browne H, Mason G, Tang T. Retinoids and pregnancy: an update. The Obstetrician & Gynaecologist 2014;16:7–11.

The incidence of spontaneous miscarriage is considered to be 20–40%.

The overall risks of fetal malformations in live born infants exposed to isotretinoin in utero are estimated to be 20–35%.

324 A woman presents at 8 weeks gestation in her first pregnancy with severe nausea and vomiting of pregnancy (NVP). Her thyroid function test (TFT) results are as follows:

TSH: 0.1 mU/l

FT4: 20 pmol/l

What is the most appropriate management plan?

A. Commence carbimazole and check TSH receptor antibodies

B. Commence propylthiouracil (PTU) and repeat TFT in 6 weeks

C. **Supportive treatment for NVP and check TSH receptor antibodies**

D. Supportive treatment for NVP and repeat TFT in 6 weeks

E. Supportive treatment for NVP only

TOG Article

Jefferys A, Vanderpump M, Yasmin E. Thyroid dysfunction and reproductive health. The Obstetrician & Gynaecologist 2015;17:39–45.

Graves' disease presenting in pregnancy can be difficult to differentiate from gestational hyperthyroidism, which affects 1–3% of pregnancies and occurs because of stimulation of TSH receptors by Beta human chorionic gonadotropin (βHCG). Free T4 levels are raised in both conditions but TSH receptor antibodies are usually positive and diagnostic of Graves' disease. As free T4 levels tend to return to normal in the second trimester, supportive management is generally sufficient in gestational hyperthyroidism and antithyroid medication is not usually required.

325 A 30-year-old woman visits her GP at 8 weeks gestation in her second pregnancy with mild symptoms of NVP. She had severe NVP in her first pregnancy requiring hospital admission and is concerned that her symptoms will worsen.

What is the most appropriate advice from her GP?

A. Admission to hospital for assessment and treatment

B. Outpatient hospital attendance for intravenous rehydration

C. Reassurance that severe NVP is unlikely to recur

D. Treatment with cyclizine if symptoms worsen

E. Treatment with ondansetron if symptoms worsen

TOG Article

Gadsby R, Barnie-Adshead T. Severe nausea and vomiting of pregnancy: should it be treated with appropriate pharmacotherapy? The Obstetrician & Gynaecologist 2011;13:107–111.

An antenatal guideline published by the National Institute for Health and Clinical Excellence (NICE) in June 2008 states that if a woman requests or would like to consider treatment for NVP, antihistamines should be used. This is the only pharmacological treatment for NVP mentioned in the recommendation section.

326 What percentage of pregnant women with hyperemesis gravidarum in early pregnancy experience transient hyperthyroidism?

A. 20%

B. 30%

C. 40%

D. 50%

E. 60%

Journal Article

Jarvis S. Management of nausea and vomiting in pregnancy BMJ 2011;342.

One prospective study found evidence of transient hyperthyroidism in 60% of women with hyperemesis gravidarum. The degree of hyperthyroidism and HCG concentrations correlate with the severity of vomiting and in most women thyroid dysfunction is self-limiting. Higher concentrations of progesterone, adrenocorticotrophic hormone and leptin have also been associated with hyperemesis.

327 A 26-year-old patient presents with left iliac fossa pain and has a 6 week period of amenorrhoea. The patient is clinically stable. An ultrasound confirms the presence of a left-sided ectopic pregnancy. There is a 2x2x2 cm pool of free fluid in the pouch of Douglas and the serum βHCG level is 3500 IU/l.

What is the recommended management?

A. Left Laparoscopic salpingectomy, if the contralateral tube is healthy

B. Left Laparoscopic Salpingotomy

C. Left Salpingectomy via a laparotomy

D. Methotrexate

E. Repeat the βHCG levels and manage accordingly

GTG 21 The Management of Tubal Pregnancy

Methotrexate is recommended to patients who are asymptomatic, have a serum βHCG level of less than 3000 IU/l and no free fluid in the pouch of Douglas. Laparotomy is recommended in patients who are unstable and salpingotomy is recommended if the contralateral tube is healthy. A symptomatic patient with the presence of free fluid should not be managed conservatively.

328 A woman has undergone surgical management of miscarriage and a partial molar pregnancy has been confirmed. Referral to a specialist centre is advised.

Where are the three specialist referral centres in the United Kingdom?

A. Aberdeen, Birmingham, London

B. Cardiff, Edinburgh, London

C. Dundee, London, Sheffield

D. Edinburgh, London, Sheffield

E. Glasgow, London, Sheffield

GTG 38 The Management of Gestational Trophoblastic Disease

Trophoblastic Tumour Screening and Treatment Centre

Department of Medical Oncology, Charing Cross Hospital, Fulham Palace Road, London W6 8RF, Website: www.hmole-chorio.org.uk

Trophoblastic Screening and Treatment Centre

Weston Park Hospital, Whitham Road Sheffield, S10 2SJ, Website: www.chorio.group.shef.ac.uk/index.html

Hydatidiform Mole Follow-up (Scotland)

Department of Obstetrics and Gynaecology, Ninewells Hospital Dundee, DD1 9SY.

329 A woman has undergone surgical management of miscarriage and the histology confirms Gestational Trophoblastic Disease (GTD). What is the expected incidence of GTD in the United Kingdom?

A. 1 in 214 live births

B. 1 in 714 live births

C. 1 in 1254 live births

D. 1 in 2544 live births

E. 1 in 7140 live births

GTG 38 The Management of Gestational Trophoblastic Disease

GTD (hydatidiform mole, invasive mole, choriocarcinoma, placental-site trophoblastic tumor) is a rare event in the United Kingdom, with a calculated incidence of 1/714 live births.

330 A woman has been diagnosed with high-risk gestational trophoblastic neoplasia (GTN) and is about to receive multiagent chemotherapy.

What is the expected cure rate?

A. 65%

B. 75%

C. 85%

D. 95%

E. 100%

GTG 38 The Management of Gestational Trophoblastic Disease

In the United Kingdom, there exists an effective registration and treatment programme.

The programme has achieved impressive results.

The cure rate for women with a score of ≤ 6 is almost 100%; the rate for women with a score of ≥ 7 is 95%

331 A woman has attended the gynaecology clinic to discuss a diagnosis of a molar pregnancy.

What is the definitive method of diagnosis?

A. Clinical assessment

B. Histologic analysis of tissue

C. Serum βHCG levels

D. Ultrasound

E. Urine βHCG levels

GTG 38 The Management of Gestational Trophoblastic Disease

Ultrasound examination is helpful in making a pre-evacuation diagnosis but the definitive diagnosis is made by histologic examination of the products of conception.

332 A woman underwent medical management of miscarriage but no specimen was sent for histological analysis.

What would be the advice to the patient following this procedure?

A. Do nothing

B. If your period does not return within 6 weeks do a home pregnancy test

C. Perform a home pregnancy test in 1 week

D. Perform a home pregnancy test in 3 weeks

E. Perform a home pregnancy test in 5 weeks

GTG 38 The Management of Gestational Trophoblastic Disease

A urinary pregnancy test should be performed 3 weeks after medical management of a failed pregnancy if products of conception are not sent for histological examination.

333 During a routine surgical evacuation of miscarriage when should oxytocic agents be used?

A. Always

B. If blood loss exceeds 50 ml

C. If blood loss exceeds 150 ml

D. If blood loss exceeds 250 ml

E. If life-threatening bleeding is encountered

GTG 38 The Management of Gestational Trophoblastic Disease

Excessive vaginal bleeding can be associated with molar pregnancy and consultation with a senior surgeon directly supervising surgical evacuation is advised.

The use of oxytocic infusion prior to completion of the evacuation is not recommended.

If the woman is experiencing significant haemorrhage prior to evacuation, surgical evacuation should be expedited and the need for oxytocin infusion weighed up against the risk of tumor embolisation. Excessive vaginal bleeding can be associated with molar pregnancy.

Theoretical evidence raises concern over the routine use of potent oxytocic agents because of its potential to embolise and disseminate trophoblastic tissue through the venous system.

To control life-threatening bleeding, oxytocic infusions may be used.

334 A woman has had surgical management of miscarriage and a molar pregnancy has been confirmed.

Which immunohistochemistry marker is useful for distinguishing between partial and complete molar pregnancies?

A. P16

B. P53

C. P57

D. P87

E. P96

GTG 38 The Management of Gestational Trophoblastic Disease

Ploidy status and immunohistochemistry staining for P57 may help in distinguishing partial from complete moles.

335 A woman has had an ultrasound scan and the possibility of a molar pregnancy with a co-existing twin has been raised by the sonographer.

The woman has been referred to a regional fetal medicine centre for further investigations.

What would be the most appropriate investigation?

A. Fetal blood sampling for βHCG levels of the suspected molar pregnancy

B. Karyotyping of the suspected molar pregnancy

C. Karyotyping of the mother

D. MRI scan

E. Serum βHCG levels

GTG 38 The Management of Gestational Trophoblastic Disease

When there is diagnostic doubt about the possibility of a combined molar pregnancy with a viable, advice should be sought from the regional fetal medicine unit and the relevant trophoblastic screening centre.

In the situation of a twin pregnancy where there is one viable fetus and the other pregnancy is molar, the woman should be counselled about the increased risk of perinatal morbidity and outcome for GTN.

Prenatal invasive testing for fetal karyotype should be considered in cases where it is unclear if the pregnancy is a complete mole with a coexisting normal twin or a partial mole.

Prenatal invasive testing for fetal karyotype should also be considered in cases of abnormal placenta, such as suspected mesenchymal hyperplasia of the placenta.

336 What percentage of partial molar pregnancies consist of tetraploid or mosaic conceptions?

A. 10%

B. 25%

C. 50%

D. 75%

E. 90%

GTG 38 The Management of Gestational Trophoblastic Disease

Partial moles are usually (90%) triploid in origin, with two sets of paternal haploid genes and one set of maternal haploid genes. Partial moles occur, in almost all cases, following dispermic fertilisation of an ovum.

Ten percent of partial moles represent tetraploid or mosaic conceptions. In a partial mole, there is usually evidence of a fetus or fetal red blood cells.

337 A 25-year-old woman attends the Early Pregnancy Unit with vomiting and bleeding. An ultrasound scan is performed, which is strongly suggestive of a molar pregnancy.

What is the optimal method of uterine evacuation?

A. Medical evacuation with Methotrexate

B. Medical evacuation with Mifepristone and Misoprostol

C. Medical Evacuation with Oxytocin

D. Suction curettage

E. Total Hysterectomy

GTG 38 The Management of Gestational Trophoblastic Disease

Complete molar pregnancies are not associated with fetal parts, therefore suction evacuation is the method of choice for uterine evacuation.

Medical evacuation of complete molar pregnancies should be avoided if possible.

Data on the management of molar pregnancies with mifepristone and misoprostol are limited.

338 A 30-year-old woman attends the preconception counselling clinic. She has completed follow-up with the regional trophoblastic screening centre following a partial molar pregnancy.

She is keen to try and conceive again, but wishes to know the risk of a further molar pregnancy.

What would you tell her the risk is?

A. 1/10

B. 1/25

C. 1/50

D. 1/80

E. 1/200

GTG 38 The Management of Gestational Trophoblastic Disease

Women should be advised not to conceive until their follow-up is complete.

The risk of a further molar pregnancy is low (1/80): more than 98% of women who become pregnant following a molar pregnancy will neither have a further molar pregnancy nor are they at increased risk of obstetric complications.

339 A woman attends the early pregnancy unit having experienced her second successive miscarriage.

She has been researching miscarriage on the internet and has read that most miscarriages are due to genetic problems.

What percentage of first-trimester miscarriages are due to chromosomal abnormalities?

A. 50%

B. 60%

C. 70%

D. 80%

E. 90%

TOG Article

Morley L, Shillito J, Tang T. Preventing recurrent miscarriage of unknown aetiology. The Obstetrician & Gynaecologist 2013;15:99–105.

Chromosomal abnormalities are considered to account for 70% of sporadic first trimester miscarriages.

340 What is the age-related risk of miscarriage in women under 20 years of age?

A. 5%

B. 13%

C. 20%

D. 28%

E. 35%

GTG 17 The Investigation and Treatment of Couples with Recurrent First trimester and Second-Trimester Miscarriage

Maternal age and number of previous miscarriages are two independent risk factors for a further miscarriage.

Advancing maternal age is associated with a decline in both the number and quality of the remaining oocytes. A large prospective register linkage study reported the age-related risk of miscarriage in recognised pregnancies to be:

13% in 12–19 years

11% in 20–24 years

12% in 25–29 years 15% in 30–34 years

25% in 35–39 years

51% in 40–44 years

93% in ≥45 years

341 A woman attends the miscarriage clinic having experienced her third consecutive first-trimester loss.

Which investigations should be undertaken?

	Investigation					
Antiphospholipid antibodies	Karyotyping of both parents	Pelvic ultrasound scan	Thrombophilia screen	Cytogenetics of products of conception	Maternal peripheral natural killer cells	TORCH screen
A. X	X		X		X	
B. X		X	X	X		
C. X	X				X	X
D.	X	X	X			X
E. X	X			X		

GTG 17 The Investigation and Treatment of Couples with Recurrent First trimester and Second-Trimester Miscarriage

All women with recurrent first-trimester miscarriage and all women with one or more second-trimester miscarriage should be screened before pregnancy for antiphospholipid antibodies.

Cytogenetic analysis should be performed on products of conception of the third and subsequent consecutive miscarriage(s).

Parental peripheral blood karyotyping of both partners should be performed in couples with recurrent miscarriage where testing of products of conception reports an unbalanced structural chromosomal abnormality.

All women with recurrent first-trimester miscarriage and all women with one or more second-trimester miscarriages should have a pelvic ultrasound to assess uterine anatomy.

Suspected uterine anomalies may require further investigations to confirm the diagnosis, using hysteroscopy, laparoscopy or three-dimensional pelvic ultrasound.

Women with second-trimester miscarriage should be screened for inherited thrombophilias including factor V Leiden, factor II (prothrombin) gene mutation and protein S.

342 Which B vitamin has been shown to be effective in the reduction of nausea and vomiting of pregnancy (NVP)?

    A. Cobalamin
    B. Folic acid
    C. Pyridoxine
    D. Riboflavin
    E. Thiamine

TOG Article

Gadsby R, Barnie-Adshead T. Severe nausea and vomiting of pregnancy: should it be treated with appropriate pharmacotherapy? The Obstetrician & Gynaecologist 2011;13:107–111.

There is evidence that pyridoxine is effective in treating NVP. In one randomised controlled trial, 59 pregnant women received either 25 mg pyridoxine or placebo three times a day: in the pyridoxine group there was a significant reduction in the mean nausea score and in the number of participants with vomiting.

343 A 30-year-old woman attends the early pregnancy unit with a positive pregnancy test and some lower abdominal pain. Her last menstrual period was approximately 8 weeks ago, but her menstrual cycle is irregular.

A transvaginal ultrasound scan is organised, which demonstrates an intrauterine gestation sac with fetal pole and yolk sac, but no fetal heartbeat is identified. The crown-rump length (CRL) is 6 mm.

What is the correct course of action?

A. Inform the woman that she has a missed miscarriage and arrange surgical evacuation

B. Inform the woman that she has a missed miscarriage and arrange medical evacuation with misoprostol

C. Inform the woman that she has a missed miscarriage and arrange medical evacuation with mifepristone and misoprostol

D. Inform the woman that the pregnancy appears normal and no further intervention is required

E. Inform the woman that the viability of the pregnancy is uncertain and arrange for a further scan in 7–10 days

NICE CG 154 Ectopic Pregnancy and Miscarriage

If the CRL is less than 7.0 mm with a transvaginal ultrasound scan and there is no visible heartbeat, perform a second scan a minimum of 7 days after the first before making a diagnosis. Further scans may be needed before a diagnosis can be made.

344 A woman who has had a left salpingectomy previously for ectopic pregnancy has now been diagnosed with an ectopic pregnancy in the right fallopian tube.

A laparoscopy is performed and the surgeon opts for a salpingo-tomy as the woman still wishes to become pregnant.

What is the possibility that she will require further treatment (methotrexate or salpingectomy)?

A. 1%

B. 5%

C. 10%

D. 20%

E. 50%

NICE CG 154 Ectopic Pregnancy and Miscarriage

Women having a salpingotomy should be informed that up to 1 in 5 women may need further treatment. This treatment may include methotrexate and/or a salpingectomy.

345 A woman attends the early pregnancy unit and has a confirmed diagnosis of miscarriage. She is fit and well, and all observations are normal.

What is the recommended first line management?

A. Evacuation of retained products of conception

B. Expectant management for 7–14 days

C. Intramuscular Methotrexate

D. Oral Mifepristone

E. Vaginal Misoprostol

NICE CG 154 Ectopic Pregnancy and Miscarriage

Use expectant management for 7–14 days as the first-line management strategy for women with a confirmed diagnosis of miscarriage.

346 A woman who has blood group A Rh negative undergoes a laparo-scopic salpingectomy for a ruptured ectopic pregnancy.

What anti-D rhesus prophylaxis is required?

A. 250 IU anti-D

B. 500 IU anti-D

C. Two doses of 250 IU anti-D 48 hours apart

D. No prophylaxis required

E. Quantify the feto-maternal haemorrhage with a Kleihauer test to determine the correct dose of anti-D

NICE CG 154 Ectopic Pregnancy and Miscarriage

Offer anti-D rhesus prophylaxis at a dose of 250 IU (50 micrograms) to all rhesus negative women who undergo a surgical procedure to manage an ectopic pregnancy or a miscarriage.

347 A woman underwent a surgical evacuation of the uterus following a failed intrauterine pregnancy.

The products of conception were sent for histological analysis and a diagnosis of complete molar pregnancy was made.

The woman was referred to the regional trophoblastic disease centre for follow-up, and subsequently required treatment with single-agent chemotherapy.

She returns to clinic after completion of treatment as she wishes to conceive again.

How long should she wait?

A. 1 month

B. 3 months

C. 6 months

D. 12 months

E. 18 months

GTG 38 The Management of Gestational Trophoblastic Disease

Women should be advised not to conceive until their follow-up is complete.

Women who undergo chemotherapy are advised not to conceive for 1 year after completion of treatment.

348 A woman attends for her first trimester dating scan at 12 weeks gestation and all appears well. Both fetal heart and fetal movements are seen.

What is the chance that she will miscarry before 24 weeks of gestation?

A. 0.1–0.2%
B. 0.5–0.6%
C. 1–2%
D. 5–6%
E. 10–15%

GTG 17 The Investigation and Treatment of Couples with Recurrent First-trimester and Second-Trimester Miscarriage

It has been estimated that 1–2% of second-trimester pregnancies miscarry before 24 weeks of gestation.

349 What investigation is indicated for women following a second-trimester miscarriage, which is not indicated in recurrent first-trimester loss?

A. Anticardiolipin antibodies
B. Karyotyping of products of conception
C. Lupus anticoagulant
D. Pelvic ultrasound scan
E. **Thrombophilia screen**

GTG 17 The Investigation and Treatment of Couples with Recurrent First-trimester and Second-Trimester Miscarriage

Women with second-trimester miscarriage should be screened for inherited thrombophilias including factor V Leiden, factor II (prothrombin) gene mutation and protein S.

350 A healthy 30-year-old woman with recurrent first-trimester miscarriage attends the clinic for investigation and all tests recommended in the RCOG guideline are reported as normal.

The woman is a member of an internet support group for miscarriage and has heard from other members that there may be other adjunctive treatments that can be used.

What treatment would you recommend?

A. HCG supplementation

B. Immunoglobulin intravenously

C. **No adjunctive treatment of proven benefit in this situation**

D. Paternal white cell transfusion

E. Progesterone supplementation

GTG 17 The Investigation and Treatment of Couples with Recurrent First-trimester and Second-Trimester Miscarriage

There is insufficient evidence to evaluate the effect of progesterone supplementation in pregnancy to prevent a miscarriage in women with recurrent miscarriage.

There is insufficient evidence to evaluate the effect of human chorionic gonadotrophin supplementation in pregnancy to prevent a miscarriage in women with recurrent miscarriage.

Paternal cell immunisation, third-party donor leucocytes, trophoblast membranes and intravenous immunoglobulin in women with previous unexplained recurrent miscarriage do not improve the live birth rate.

Module 17

Gynaecological Oncology

351 Administration of tamoxifen is a cornerstone in the treatment of breast cancer, but it has a weak estrogenic effect on the endometrium.

A woman who is taking Tamoxifen presents with post-menopausal bleeding (PMB).

What is her risk of developing endometrial cancer when compared to the general population?

A. No increased risk

B. 1–2 times

C. 3–6 times

D. 8–10 times

E. 15–20 times

TOG Article

Bakour SH, Timmermans A, Mol BW, Khan KS. Management of women with postmenopausal bleeding: evidence-based review. The Obstetrician & Gynaecologist 2012;14:243–249.

Administeration of tamoxifen is a cornerstone in the treatment of breast cancer. Women receiving tamoxifen experience a three- to six-fold greater incidence of endometrial cancer due to its weak estrogenic effect on the endometrium. The presentation of PMB therefore requires urgent investigation in this group of women. Treatment beyond 5 years increases the risk by at least four-fold.

352 PMB is defined as uterine bleeding occurring after at least one year of amenorrhoea. The main purpose of investigating a woman with PMB is to rule out endometrial cancer.

Part 2 MRCOG: Single Best Answer Questions, First Edition.
Andrew Sizer, Chandrika Balachandar, Nibedan Biswas, Richard Foon,
Anthony Griffiths, Sheena Hodgett, Banchhita Sahu and Martyn Underwood.

What is the risk that a women presenting with PMB will have endometrial cancer?

A. 5–10%

B. 10–15%

C. 15–20%

D. 20–25%

E. 25–30%

TOG Article

Bakour SH, Timmermans A, Mol BW, Khan KS. Management of women with postmenopausal bleeding: evidence-based review. The Obstetrician & Gynaecologist 2012;14:243–249.

PMB, defined as uterine bleeding occurring after at least 1 year of amenorrhoea, is a common clinical condition with an incidence of 10% immediately after menopause. Patients with PMB have a 10–15% chance of having endometrial carcinoma.

353 A 60-year-old woman presents with a first episode of PMB.
What is the most appropriate first line of investigation?

A. Dilatation and Curettage to assess the endometrium

B. Hysteroscopy to assess the endometrial cavity and obtain an endometrial sample

C. Pipelle biopsy to obtain an endometrial sample

D. Saline infusion sonography to measure the endometrial thickness

E. Transvaginal sonography to assess the endometrial thickness

TOG Article

Bakour SH, Timmermans A, Mol BW, Khan KS. Management of women with postmenopausal bleeding: evidence-based review. The Obstetrician & Gynaecologist 2012;14:243–249.

The relatively noninvasive nature of TVS makes it more acceptable, especially to older women. The mean endometrial thickness in postmenopausal women is much thinner than in premenopausal women. The likelihood of important pathology (cancer) being present increases with increasing thickness of the endometrium.

The meta-analysis by Smith–Bindman et al. included 5892 women from 35 prospective studies that compared endometrial thickness measured at TVS to the presence or absence of endometrial carcinoma on histology. At ≤5 mm cut-off, the overall summary of mean-weighted estimates of the sensitivity for detecting endometrial cancer was 96%

for a 39% false-positive rate. This would reduce a pretest probability of 10% for endometrial cancer to a post-test probability of 1%.

354 A 55-year-old woman presents with a first episode of PMB. A transvaginal ultrasound scan showed an endometrial thickness of 3.8mm.

What is the most appropriate management plan?

A. Book a repeat transvaginal scan in 6 months

B. Book for an out-patient hysteroscopy to look at endometrial cavity and obtain endometrial sample

C. Perform a dilatation and curettage

D. Perform an endometrial sampling to rule out endometrial cancer

E. Reassure, follow expectant management

TOG Article

Bakour SH, Timmermans A, Mol BW, Khan KS. Management of women with postmenopausal bleeding: evidence-based review. The Obstetrician & Gynaecologist 2012;14:243–249.

Study by Gull B et al. (2000) showed that none of the woman with PMB with endometrial thickness <4 mm on transvaginal scan on expectant management developed cancer in over 1 year of follow-up.

355 A 60 year old undergoes hysterectomy and bilateral salpingo-oophorectomy for grade 1 endometrial cancer.

The final histology report confirms tumor invading the uterine serosa.

As per the new FIGO staging of endometrial cancer, what is the stage?

A. Stage IC

B. Stage IIC

C. Stage IIIA

D. Stage IIIB

E. Stage IIIC

Journal Article

Pecorelli S. Revised FIGO staging for carcinoma of the vulva, cervix, and endometrium. International Journal of Gynaecology & Obstetrics 2009;105:103–104.

    II Cervical stromal invasion, but not beyond uterus

    IIIA Tumor invades serosa or adnexa

    IIIB Vaginal and/or parametrial involvement

    IIIC1 Pelvic node involvement

    IIIC2 Para-aortic involvement.

356 Ovarian cysts are common in postmenopausal women, although their prevalence is lower than in premenopausal women.

A 59-year-old woman is referred to the clinic with fullness in the lower abdomen and a serum CA125 level of 64iu/l.

What is the first line of investigation?

A. Computed Tomography (CT) of abdomen and pelvis

B. MRI of pelvis

C. PET scan

D. Transvaginal ultrasound scan of pelvis

E. USS of pelvis with Doppler

GTG 34 Ovarian Cysts in Postmenopausal Women

It is recommended that ovarian cysts in postmenopausal women should be assessed using CA125 and transvaginal grey scale sonography. There is no routine role yet for Doppler, MRI, CT or PET.

357 It is recommended that 'risk of malignancy index' (RMI) should be used to triage post-menopausal women with an ovarian cyst to assess low, moderate or high risk of malignancy.

This is calculated as U (ultrasound score) X M (menopausal status) X CA125.

What is the RMI of a post-menopausal woman with a CA125 of 15, ultrasound showing 6 cm bilateral, multiloculated cyst?

A. 45

B. 90

C. 95

D. 130

E. 135

GTG 34 Ovarian Cysts in Postmenopausal Women
RMI = U × M × CA125

$U = 0$ (for ultrasound score of 0); $U = 1$ (for ultrasound score of 1); $U = 3$ (for ultrasound score of 2–5).

Ultrasound scans are scored one point for each of the following characteristics: multilocular cyst; evidence of solid areas; evidence of metastases; presence of ascites; bilateral lesions.

$M = 3$ for all postmenopausal women 1 for premenopausal women.

CA125 is serum CA125 measurement in u/ml.

358 It is recommended that RMI should be used to triage post-menopausal women with ovarian cyst to assess low, moderate or high risk of malignancy.

This is calculated as U (ultrasound score) × M (menopausal status) × CA125.

What is the risk of ovarian cancer in a woman who has an RMI of 25–250 (moderate risk)?

A. 3%

B. 20%

C. 25%

D. 60%

E. 75%

GTG 34 Ovarian Cysts in Postmenopausal Women

Women with an RMI of <25 have low risk of developing ovarian cancer (<3%).

Women with an RMI of 25–250 have moderate risk of developing ovarian cancer (20%).

Women with an RMI of >250 have high risk of developing ovarian cancer (75%).

359 Who should be responsible for the management of women with intermediate risk of malignancy (RMI of 25–250)?

A. General gynaecologist in a cancer centre

B. General gynaecologist in a cancer unit

C. General gynaecologist in a district general hospital

D. Gynaecological oncologist in a cancer centre

E. Lead clinician in a cancer unit

GTG 34 Ovarian Cysts in Postmenopausal Women

Women need to be triaged, so that a gynaecological oncologist in a cancer centre operates on those at high risk of having ovarian cancer, a lead clinician in a cancer unit operates on those at moderate risk, while those at low risk may be operated on by a general gynaecologist or offered conservative management.

360 Borderline ovarian tumors are a distinct pathological group of neoplasms typically seen in younger women. They are often diagnosed at an earlier stage resulting in excellent prognosis.

What is the histologic feature that differentiates borderline ovarian tumors from invasive ovarian cancers?

A. Absence of hyperchromasia

B. Absence of stromal invasion

C. Presence of extra ovarian invasive implants

D. Presence of mitotic figures

E. Presence of prominent nucleoli

Bagade P, Edmondson R, Nayar A. Management of borderline ovarian tumours. The Obstetrician & Gynaecologist 2012;14:115–120.

A histologic feature of borderline ovarian tumors includes nuclear stratification and hyperchromasia and the presence of mitotic figures and prominent nucleoli. Stromal invasion is absent, which distinguishes them from invasive carcinomas.

361 A 49-year-old para 3 underwent laparoscopic left salpingo-oophorectomy for a complex left ovarian cyst. Histology shows a serous micro papillary borderline ovarian tumor with the presence of DNA aneuploidy.

What is the most appropriate management plan?

A. CT scan in 6 months time

B. Reassure and discharge

C. Right salpingo-oophorectomy

D. Total abdominal hysterectomy and right salpingo-oophorectomy

E. Total abdominal hysterectomy and right salpingo-oophorectomy, peritoneal washings, infracolic omentectomy and exploration of entire abdominal cavity

TOG Article

Bagade P, Edmondson R, Nayar A. Management of borderline ovarian tumours. The Obstetrician & Gynaecologist 2012;14:115–120.

An older woman with no fertility concerns who had limited assessment during primary surgery should undergo complete staging, which includes total abdominal hysterectomy and bilateral salpingo-oophorectomy, peritoneal washings, infracolic omentectomy and exploration of entire abdominal cavity. Presence of DNA aneuploidy is associated with 19-fold increase with the subsequent risk of dying.

362 Borderline ovarian tumors are also known as tumors of low malignant potential. They constitute 10–15% of all epithelial ovarian neoplasms.

What is the 5-year survival rate of stage 1 borderline ovarian tumor?

A. 75–77%

B. 80–83%

C. 85–87%

D. 90–93%

E. 95–97%

TOG Article

Bagade P, Edmondson R, Nayar A. Management of borderline ovarian tumours. The Obstetrician & Gynaecologist 2012;14:115–120.

The 5-year survival rate of stage 1 borderline ovarian tumor varies from 95–97%. Even women with stage III disease have a good prognosis with a survival rate of 50–86%.

363 The lifetime risk of ovarian cancer in the general population is 1.4%. However, women with hereditary ovarian cancer syndrome have significantly higher risks of developing ovarian cancer.

What is the risk of ovarian cancer in a woman who has a BRCA1 mutation carrier?

A. 15–25%

B. 25–35%

C. 35–45%

D. 45–55%

E. 55–65%

TOG Article

Gaughan EMG, Walsh TA. Risk-reducing surgery for women at high risk of epithelial ovarian cancer. The Obstetrician & Gynaecologist 2014;16:185–191.

BRCA mutations account for up to 90% of hereditary ovarian cancer. The estimated risk of ovarian cancer is 35–46% for a BRCA1 mutation carrier and 13–23% for a BRCA2 mutation carrier.

364 Lynch syndrome, also called hereditary nonpolyposis colorectal cancer (HNPCC) is associated with the development of multiple types of cancer.

What is the suggested management for reduction of risk of developing gynaecological cancers in a 35-year-old woman with HNPCC who has completed her family?

A. 6 monthly CA125 and transvaginal ultrasound

B. 12 monthly CA125 and transvaginal ultrasound

C. Hysterectomy and bilateral salpingo-oophorectomy

D. Laparoscopic bilateral salpingo-oophorectomy

E. Regular use of combined oral contraceptive pills

TOG Article

Gaughan EMG, Walsh TA. Risk-reducing surgery for women at high risk of epithelial ovarian cancer. The Obstetrician & Gynaecologist 2014;16:185–191.

HNPCC is associated with cancer diagnosis at an early age and the development of multiple cancer types, particularly colon and endometrial cancer. They have a 3–14% risk of developing ovarian cancer.

365 NICE recommends not to include systematic retroperitoneal lymphadenectomy as part of standard surgical treatment in women with suspected ovarian cancer whose disease appears to be confined to the ovaries (that is, who appears to have stage I disease). What is systematic retroperitoneal lymphadenectomy?

A. Block dissection of common, external and internal iliac and obturator lymph nodes

B. Block dissection of common, external and internal iliac lymph nodes

C. Block dissection of common, external and internal iliac, obturator, lower para-aortic and bifurcation of aorta lymph nodes

D. Block dissection of lymph nodes from the pelvic side walls to the level of the renal veins)

E. Block dissection of the para-aortic lymph nodes

NICE CG 122 Ovarian cancer: The recognition and initial management of ovarian cancer.

Systematic lymphadenectomy is defined here as the removal of lymph nodes in specific areas including the upper para-aortic region above the inferior mesenteric artery (IMA), the lower para-aortic region between the IMA and the bifurcation of the aorta, the inter-aortocaval area, the right paracaval area, the common and external iliac vessels, the obturator fossa and the internal iliac vessels

366 NICE recommends that women with suspected stage 1 ovarian cancer should undergo optimal surgical staging.
What is optimal surgical staging?

A. Midline laparotomy to allow thorough assessment of the abdomen and pelvis; a total abdominal hysterectomy, bilateral salpingo-oophorectomy and infracolic omentectomy; biopsies of any peritoneal deposits; random biopsies of the pelvic and abdominal peritoneum; and retroperitoneal lymph node assessment

B. Midline laparotomy to allow thorough assessment of the abdomen and pelvis; a total abdominal hysterectomy, bilateral salpingo-oophorectomy and infracolic omentectomy and retroperitoneal lymph node assessment

C. Midline laparotomy to allow thorough assessment of the abdomen and pelvis; a total abdominal hysterectomy, bilateral salpingo-oophorectomy and infracolic omentectomy; biopsies of any peritoneal deposits; random biopsies of the pelvic and abdominal peritoneum

D. Midline laparotomy to allow thorough assessment of the abdomen and pelvis; a total abdominal hysterectomy, bilateral salpingo-oophorectomy and infracolic omental biopsy; biopsies of any peritoneal deposits; random biopsies of the pelvic and abdominal peritoneum; and retroperitoneal lymph node assessment

E. Midline laparotomy to allow thorough assessment of the abdomen and pelvis; a total abdominal hysterectomy, bilateral salpingo-oophorectomy and infracolic omentectomy; biopsies of any peritoneal deposits; random biopsies of the pelvic and abdominal peritoneum; and systematic retroperitoneal lymphadenectomy

NICE CG 122 Ovarian cancer: The recognition and initial management of ovarian cancer.

As above

367 A 70-year-old woman underwent optimal surgical staging for suspected early stage ovarian cancer. Her final histology showed stage 1a grade 3 epithelial ovarian cancers.

What is the preferred plan of care after discussion in MDT?

A. Follow-up in 3 months with CT scan and serum Ca125

B. Follow-up in 6 months with CT scan and serum Ca125

C. Offer adjuvant Chemotherapy as 6 cycles of Carboplatin

D. Offer adjuvant Chemotherapy as 6 Cycles of Carboplatin and Bevacizumab

E. Offer adjuvant Chemotherapy as 6 Cycles of Carboplatin and Taxol

NICE CG 122 Ovarian cancer: The recognition and initial management of ovarian cancer.

Offer women with high-risk stage I disease (grade 3 or stage Ic) adjuvant chemotherapy consisting of six cycles of carboplatin.

368 It is estimated that 75% of women with ovarian cancer currently receive a paclitaxel/platinum combination as first-line therapy.

Although most patients (70–80%) initially respond to first-line chemotherapy, most responders eventually relapse (55–75% within 2 years).

What is the definition of 'Complete response' to chemotherapy?

A. Malignant disease not detectable for at least 4 weeks

B. Malignant disease not detectable for at least 8 weeks

C. Malignant disease not detectable for at least 12 weeks

D. Malignant disease not detectable for at least 6 months

E. Malignant disease not detectable for at least 12 months

NICE TA 55 Guidance on the use of paclitaxel in the treatment of ovarian cancer.

A complete response is defined as malignant disease not detectable for at least 4 weeks, and a partial response is defined as tumor size reduced by at least 50% for more than 4 weeks.

369 A 70-year-old woman has undergone laparotomy for suspected ovarian cancer. At laparotomy, the cancer is found to involve the left ovary and uterus and she has positive peritoneal washings.

As per the FIGO classification for staging of ovarian cancer, what is her staging?

A. Stage IC

B. Stage IIA

C. Stage IIB

D. Stage IIC

E. Stage IIIC

Journal Article

Prat J. FIGO Committee on Gynecologic Oncology. Staging classification for cancer of the ovary, fallopian tube, and peritoneum. International Journal of Gynaecology & Obstetrics 2014;124:1–5.

In stage II, cancer is diagnosed in one or both ovaries and has spread into other areas of the pelvis.

- Stage IIA: Cancer has spread to the uterus and/or the fallopian tubes.
- Stage IIB: Cancer has spread to other tissue within the pelvis.
- Stage IIC: Cancer is diagnosed in one or both ovaries and has spread to the uterus and/or fallopian tubes, or to other tissue within the pelvis. Also, one of the following is true:
  - cancer is also diagnosed on the outside surface of one or both ovaries; or
  - the capsule of the ovary has ruptured; or
  - positive peritoneal washings

370 A 65-year-old woman complaining of severe itching is diagnosed with Vulval intraepithelial neoplasia (VIN) 3 on biopsy.

What is the first line of management?

A. Laser ablation

B. Local excision

C. Topical cidofir

D. Topical imiquimod

E. Wait and watch

GTG 58 Management of vulval skin disorders

Women undergo treatment of VIN to relieve symptoms of severe pruritus, to exclude invasive disease and to reduce the risk of developing invasive cancer.

371 A 65-year-old woman presents with a history of vulval discomfort and soreness for 6 months. On examination, there is 2.5 cm raised ulcerated area on the left labia majora which looks highly suspicious of vulval cancer.

What is the first line of investigation?

A. Multiple punch biopsies with adjacent normal skin

B. Sentinel lymph node biopsy

C. Urgent CT scan

D. Urgent MRI

E. Wide local excision biopsy

TOG Article

Bailey C, Luesley D. Squamous vulval cancer–an update. The Obstetrician & Gynaecologist 2013;15:227–231.

Diagnosis of Vulval cancer is made by punch biopsy of the suspicious area. Wide excision biopsy should be avoided as if the initial lesion is absent and the women needs further excision, it can be extremely challenging to ensure a good clearance margin of at least 1 cm.

372 In vulval cancer, the depth of invasion directly correlates with lymph node involvement, thus affecting prognosis and the management plan.

What is the rate of lymph node involvement in women with stage 1a (<1mm invasion) vulval cancer?

A. <1%

B. 5%

C. 7.5%

D. 10%

E. 25%

Bailey C, Luesley D. Squamous vulval cancer–an update. The Obstetrician & Gynaecologist 2013;15:227–231.

Vulval tumors with <1mm invasion (stage 1a) also known as superficially invasive squamous cancers have a negligible risk of lymph node metastasis; thus, the need for nodal resection is eliminated in these cases.

373 Vulval cancers are relatively rare cancers with surgery as the mainstay of treatment. In recent years, a lot of emphasis has been given to sentinel node biopsy to decide management.

What is the role of sentinel node biopsy in the management of early vulval cancer?

A. To decide interval of follow-up

B. To decide on the need for lymph node resection

C. To decide on the need for postoperative radiotherapy

D. To evaluate for postoperative chemo radiotherapy

E. To evaluate the need for radical vulvectomy

TOG Article

Bailey C, Luesley D. Squamous vulval cancer–an update. The Obstetrician & Gynaecologist 2013;15:227–231.

The sentinel node is the node to which the tumor first drains. For women with early disease only 20% will have lymph node metastases. In a small study of 59 patients the negative predictive value of a negative sentinel lymph node was 100%. Hence, sentinel lymph node biopsy would help avoid further resection and associated complications.

374 Vulval cancers account for 6% of gynaecological cancers in the United Kingdom. In 2009, a new FIGO staging was introduced with greater emphasis on the inguino-femoral lymph node status to understand prognosis.

What is the FIGO stage for a woman who has a 3cm vulval cancer involving the anus with metastases in 2 lymph nodes <5 mm?

A. Stage IIIa

B. Stage IIIb

C. Stage IIIc

D. Stage IVa

E. Stage IVb

Journal Article
Pecorelli S, FIGO Committee on Gynecologic Oncology Revised FIGO staging for carcinoma of the vulva, cervix, and endometrium. International Journal of Gynaecology & Obstetrics 2009;105:103–104.

IIIA Tumor of any size with positive inguino-femoral lymph nodes

    (i) 1 lymph node metastasis greater than or equal to 5 mm

    (ii) 1–2 lymph node metastasis (es) of less than 5 mm

IIIB

    (i) 2 or more lymph node metastases greater than or equal to 5 mm

    (ii) 3 or more lymph node metastases less than 5 mm

IIIC Positive node(s) with extracapsular spread

375 Primary vaginal cancer is rare. There were 281 cases of vaginal cancer in the United Kingdom in 2010. The most common causes of squamous cell vaginal cancer are HPV and irradiation.
What is the most common HPV type found in vaginal cancers?
A. HPV 6
B. HPV 11
C. HPV 16
D. HPV 18
E. HPV 31

TOG Article
Lippiatt J, Powell N, Tristram A. Non-cervical human papillomavirus-related disease. The Obstetrician & Gynaecologist 2013;15:221–226.
HPV 16 is responsible for the majority of HPV-related vaginal disease.

376 Recently, the prevalence of HPV-related VIN has increased significantly and consequently the incidence of vulval cancer in young women is rising.
What are the most common HPV serotypes found in vulval cancers?
A. HPV 5 and 8
B. HPV 6 and 11
C. HPV 16 and 18
D. HPV 31 and 33
E. HPV 58 and 59

TOG Article
Bailey C, Luesley D. Squamous vulval cancer–an update. The Obstetrician & Gynaecologist 2013;15:227–231.

The vast majority of vulval cancer secondary to HPV is caused by HPV serotypes 16 and 18. A study demonstrated a 5.3-fold increase in vulval neoplasia in subjects positive for HPV-16 antibodies and in those with high antibody levels this rose 20-fold.

377 A 45-year-old woman complains of intermenstrual bleeding for the past 6 months. Past history includes 6 normal vaginal deliveries and hypertension and last smear was over 5 years ago. On speculum examination, there is a raised 2 cm friable area on the cervix.

What is the most likely diagnosis?

A. Cervical cancer
B. Cervical ectropion
C. Cervical polyp
D. Cervical warts
E. Chlamydia infection

NICE CG 27 Referral guidelines for suspected cancer.

The first symptoms of gynaecological cancer may be alterations in the menstrual cycle, intermenstrual bleeding, postcoital bleeding, PMB or vaginal discharge. When a patient presents with any of these symptoms, the primary health-care professional should undertake a full pelvic examination, including a speculum examination of the cervix.

If examination of the cervix is found to have clinical features that raise the suspicion of cervical cancer, an urgent referral should be made. A cervical smear test is not required before referral, and a previous negative cervical smear result is not a reason to delay referral.

378 A 40-year-old woman with severe dyskariosis on smear underwent colposcopy and large loop excision of transformation zone (LLETZ). Histology confirmed a moderately differentiated squamous cell carcinoma 4mm deep and 6 mm wide. Clinical and radiological examination confirmed organ confined disease.

What stage of cervical cancer is this?

A. Stage IA1
B. Stage IA2
C. Stage IB1
D. Stage IB2
E. Stage IIA1

Journal Article
Pecorelli S, FIGO Committee on Gynecologic Oncology Revised FIGO staging for carcinoma of the vulva, cervix, and endometrium. International Journal of Gynaecology & Obstetrics 2009;105:103–104.

Cervical cancer stage IA is divided into stages IA1 and IA2, based on the size of the tumor.

- In stage IA1, the cancer is not more than 3 mm deep and not more than 7 mm wide.
- In stage IA2, the cancer is more than 3 mm but not more than 5 mm deep and not more than 7 mm wide.

379 A 53-year-old woman is diagnosed with stage IA1 cervical squamous cell carcinoma after histological, clinical and radiological assessment.

What is the most appropriate management plan?

A. Conisation
B. Modified radical hysterectomy with removal of lymph nodes
C. Radical trachelectomy
D. Total abdominal hysterectomy with bilateral salpingo-oophorectomy
E. Total abdominal hysterectomy with conservation of ovaries

SIGN Guideline 99 Management of cervical cancer.
In a woman past her reproductive age the most appropriate management plan for stage IA1 Cervical Squamous cell carcinoma is total abdominal hysterectomy with bilateral salpingo-oophorectomy.

380 A 35-year-old woman is diagnosed with stage IB1 cervical squamous cell carcinoma of the cervix on histological and clinical assessment.

What is the most appropriate radiological investigation for this patient?

A. CT scan of abdomen and pelvis
B. CT scan of chest, abdomen and pelvis
C. MRI of abdomen and pelvis
D. PET CT scan
E. Ultrasound of abdomen and pelvis

SIGN Guideline 99 Management of cervical cancer.

All patients with visible, biopsy-proven cervical carcinoma (except those with FIGO IV disease) should have an MRI scan. MRI is generally superior to CT, with staging accuracy of 75–90%. The greatest value of MRI in influencing treatment options lies in the high negative predictive value for parametrial invasion (85%). Full thickness disruption of the ring of cervical stroma by tumor on MRI corresponds to FIGO stage IIB disease. Confirmation of an intact ring of cervical stroma, on adequate MRI assessment, confers potentially operable status.

Module 18

Urogynaecology and Pelvic Floor Problems

381 An 84-year-old patient who had a previous history of vaginal hysterectomy presents with a stage 3 vault prolapse. The patient has limited mobility and has previously had difficulty with the use of vaginal pessaries.

What is the most appropriate treatment option?

A. Abdominal Sacrocolpopexy

B. Colpocliesis

C. Physiotherapy

D. Sacrospinous fixation

E. Transvaginal repair with mesh

TOG Article

Ramalingam K, Monga A. Management of vault prolapse. The Obstetrician & Gynaecologist 2013;15:167.

Colpocliesis is often the procedure of choice in patients over 80 years, with a variety of comorbidities. The procedure does restore the quality of life especially in patients with limited mobility.

382 A 55-year-old patient presents with a history of urinary symptoms of urgency, increased frequency and nocturia. The patient states that she does not have symptoms of hesitancy and feels as though she empties her bladder completely.

What would be the first line of management?

A. Cystoscopy

B. Neuromodulation

C. Reduce caffeine intake and start anticholinergic medication

D. Ultrasound scan to rule out pelvic pathology

E. Urodynamics

Part 2 MRCOG: Single Best Answer Questions, First Edition.
Andrew Sizer, Chandrika Balachandar, Nibedan Biswas, Richard Foon, Anthony Griffiths, Sheena Hodgett, Banchhita Sahu and Martyn Underwood.
© 2016 John Wiley & Sons, Ltd. Published 2016 by John Wiley & Sons, Ltd.

TOG Article

Saleh S, Majumdar A, Williams K. The conservative (non-pharmacological) management of female urinary incontinence. The Obstetrician & Gynaecologist 2014;16:169–177.

It is suggested that, prior to investigating the patient, conservative treatment and medical treatment (anticholinergics) could be commenced in patients with a suspected overactive bladder.

383 A 39-year-old patient presents with symptoms of leakage of urine upon coughing, sneezing and during exercise. The symptoms started following the birth of her second child 18 months ago.

What would be the first line of management?

A. Biofeedback/Electrical stimulation

B. Bladder retraining

C. Insertion of a midurethral retropubic tape

D. Pharmacotherapy with Duloxetine

E. Supervised Pelvic floor muscle training

TOG Article

Saleh S, Majumdar A, Williams K .The conservative (non-pharmacological) management of female urinary incontinence. The Obstetrician & Gynaecologist 2014;16:169–177.

The first-line management in patients with stress incontinence is physiotherapy with pelvic floor muscle training. Bladder retraining is applicable for patients with an overactive bladder. Medical and surgical treatment would be an option if pelvic floor muscle training fails and urodynamic stress incontinence is confirmed.

384 A patient presents as an emergency with urinary retention. Upon taking a history, you also discover that the patient has been having hematuria for several weeks.

What is an absolute contraindication to inserting a suprapubic catheter?

A. Ascites

B. Bladder tumor

C. Clotting disorders

D. History of extensive bladder reconstruction

E. Unable to fill the bladder to a volume excess of 300 ml

TOG Article

Aslam N, Moran PA. Catheter use in gynaecological practice. The Obstetrician & Gynaecologist 2014;16:161–168.

An absolute contraindication to insertion of a suprapubic catheter is unexplained hematuria due to the risk of placing the catheter through the bladder tumor. All the other options are relative contraindications.

385 A 56-year-old para 4 woman presents with a vault prolapse. The patient is sexually active and urodynamic investigations fail to reveal urodynamic stress incontinence even after reduction of the prolapse.

The patient is keen on having surgery.

Which of the following operations should be offered?

A. Bilateral Sacrospinous fixation

B. Sacrocolpopexy

C. Sacrocolpopexy and insertion of a mid urethral retropubic tape

D. Sacrocolpopexy with a Burch Colposuspension

E. Unilateral Sacrospinous fixation with insertion of a mid-urethral retropubic tape

GTG 46 Post-Hysterectomy Vaginal Vault Prolapse

There is no clear evidence that the use of prophylactic continence surgery would be helpful to patients who do not have urodynamic stress incontinence. Sacrospinous fixation carries a higher risk of sexual dysfunction and Sacrospinous fixation causes more retroversion of the vagina than Sacrocolpopexy.

386 A 39-year-old para 1 patient presents with stress incontinence with no other urinary symptoms.

What would be the first line of management?

A. A trial of pelvic floor muscle training for at least 3 months

B. Electric stimulation in combination with pelvic floor muscle training

C. Pelvic floor electromyography (biofeedback)

D. Pelvic floor muscle training that involves 6 contractions done every 3 days for 6 months

E. Urodynamic studies

NICE CG 171 Urinary Incontinence: The Management of Urinary Incontinence in Women

Pelvic floor muscle training should be offered as a first-line management and should consist of eight contractions done three times weekly for at least 3 months.

387 A patient is undergoing a vaginal hysterectomy for uterine prolapse and at the end of the procedure it is noted that the vault of the vagina descends to 3 cm above the hymenal ring.

What should be considered in order to prevent further descent of the vault in the future?

A. McCall culdoplasty

B. Moschowitz-type operation

C. No further action

D. Sacrospinous fixation

E. Suturing the cardinal and uterosacral ligaments to the vaginal cuff

GTG 46 Post-Hysterectomy Vaginal Vault Prolapse

McCall culdoplasty is recommended (Grade A evidence) when compared with a Moschowitz type operation.

Suturing of the cardinal and uterosacral ligament to the vaginal cuff is evidence of grade B, and a Sacrospinous fixation is recommended if the vault descends to the end of the introitus.

388 A fit and healthy 52-year-old patient with confirmed detrusor overactivity has tried three different medical treatments (Oxybutynin, Solifenacin, Mirabegron).

The procedure that should be offered to the patient is

A. Botulinum toxin A injections into the bladder

B. Detrusor myomectomy

C. Percutaneous tibial nerve stimulation

D. Sacral nerve modulation

E. Urinary diversion

NICE CG 171 Urinary Incontinence: The Management of Urinary Incontinence in Women

After a multidisciplinary team review, patients should be offered bladder wall injection with botulinum with an overactive bladder caused by proven detrusor overactivity that has not responded to conservative management (including overactive bladder drug therapy).

389 A 38-year-old patient is suffering with stress incontinence. Her BMI is 32 kg/m^2 and the patient is interested in lifestyle management for her incontinence.

What is the most important lifestyle change that you would recommend?

A. Avoidance of caffeinated drinks
B. Exercise
C. Reduction of alcohol intake
D. Reduction of fluid intake
E. Weight loss

TOG Article

Saleh S, Majumdar A, Williams K. The conservative (non-pharmacological) management of female urinary incontinence. The Obstetrician & Gynaecologist 2014;16:169–177.

The most important conservative management for patients with stress incontinence is weight loss. Exercise is only helpful if there is associated weight loss and avoidance of caffeinated drinks and reduction in fluid intake is helpful in patients with an overactive bladder.

390 A 38-year-old patient is suffering with symptoms of an overactive bladder. Her BMI is 25 kg/m2 and the patient is interested in lifestyle changes.
What is the most important lifestyle change that you would recommend?
A. Avoidance of caffeinated drinks
B. Exercise
C. Reduction of alcohol intake
D. Reduction of fluid intake
E. Weight loss

TOG Article

Saleh S, Majumdar A, Williams K. The conservative (non-pharmacological) management of female urinary incontinence. The Obstetrician & Gynaecologist 2014;16:169–177.

There are a few randomized controlled trials demonstrating significant improvement in urinary incontinence and quality of life after following weight reduction programs. Based on a few observational studies, exercise, unless associated with weight loss, does not decrease urinary incontinence. Reduction in fluid is only weakly associated with improvement in urinary incontinence and avoidance of caffeinated drinks helps with symptoms of urgency and not stress incontinence. Large cohort studies have shown no improvement with reduction of alcohol and either stress incontinence or overactive bladder symptoms.

391 A patient presents with symptoms of a prolapse. On examination, the pelvic organ quantification score is Aa 0, Ba 0, C −5, D −7, Ap −2 Bp −2 tvl 9, gh 4, pb 3.

The patient wants her prolapse to be treated surgically.

What is the correct diagnosis and surgical treatment?

A. Stage 1 cystocele and no treatment needed

B. Stage 2 cystocele and anterior repair

C. Stage 2 rectocele and posterior repair

D. Stage 2 uterine prolapse/cystocele and vaginal hysterectomy and anterior repair

E. Stage 2 uterine prolapse/rectocele and vaginal hysterectomy and posterior repair

Journal Article

Persu C, Chapple CR, Cauni V, Gutue S, and Geavlete P. Pelvic Organ Prolapse Quantification System (POP–Q) – a new era in pelvic prolapse staging. Journal of Medicine and Life 2011;4(1):75–81.

These findings indicate that the anterior vaginal wall descends to a level of the hymen ring (stage 2 cystocele) with no significant descent of the uterus. The suggested surgical treatment is an anterior repair.

Hymen ring (distance from hymen ring cm)

	+2	+1	0	1	−2	−6		
				X				Aa
				X				Ba
						X		C
							X	D
					X			Ap
					X			Bp

C – Cervix.
D – Pouch of Douglas.
Ap/Bp – posterior vaginal wall.
Aa/Ba anterior vaginal wall.

392 A woman presents with symptoms of a prolapse. On examination, the pelvic organ quantification score is Aa −2, Ba −2, C −5, D −7, Ap 0 Bp 0 tvl 9, gh 4, pb 3

The patient wants her prolapse to be treated surgically.

What is the correct diagnosis and surgical treatment?

A. Stage 2 cystocele and anterior repair

B. Stage 1 cystocele and no treatment needed

C. Stage 2 rectocele and posterior repair

D. Stage 2 uterine prolapse/cystocele and vaginal hysterectomy and anterior repair

E. Stage 2 uterine prolapse/rectocele and vaginal hysterectomy and posterior repair

Journal Article

Persu C, Chapple CR, Cauni V, Gutue S, and Geavlete P. Pelvic Organ Prolapse Quantification System (POP–Q) – a new era in pelvic prolapse staging. J Med Life. Feb 15, 2011; 4(1): 75–81.

These findings indicate that the posterior vaginal wall descends to a level of the hymen ring (stage 2 rectocele) with no significant descent of the uterus. The suggested surgical treatment is a posterior repair.

Hymen ring (distance from hymen ring cm)

	+2	+1	0	1	−2	−6		
				X				Aa
				X				Ba
					X			C
							X	D
					X			Ap
					X			Bp

C – Cervix.
D – Pouch of Douglas.
Ap/Bp – posterior vaginal wall.
Aa/Ba anterior vaginal wall.

393 A 32-year-old multiparous woman has confirmed urodynamic stress incontinence and admits that she has not completed her family.

What management would you propose for this patient?

A. Advise the patient to compete her family before considering incontinence surgery

B. A periurethral bladder neck injection would be the treatment of choice for long-term relief

C. If the patient has had previous incontinence surgery and the incontinence recurs postpartum then await spontaneous recovery for about 3–4 months

D. If the patient has had previous incontinence surgery a Colposuspension is most likely to be safe and effective

E. If the patient insists on surgery an insertion of a midurethral retropubic tape would be the surgical treatment of choice

TOG Article

Asali F, Mahfouz I, Phillips C. The management of urogynaecological problems in pregnancy and the early postpartum period. The Obstetrician & Gynaecologist 2012; 14:153–158.

The patient should be advised to complete her family. Periurethral bulking neck injections is a useful option for short-term relief as it does not affect subsequent insertion of a midurethral retropubic tape. It is therefore a suitable option for patients who have not completed their families. If the patient has had a previous incontinence surgery and presents with recurrence postpartum they should await spontaneous recovery for 6–12 months. If the patient has had previous incontinence surgery a repeat insertion of a midurethral retropubic tape is most likely to be safe and effective.

394 A 28-year-old woman presents with a history of pelvic pain, urinary urgency, increased frequency and nocturia. The pelvic pain tends to occur during bladder filling and is relieved by voiding and you suspect that the patient has interstitial cystitis.

What other mandatory investigation is required in order to make an accurate diagnosis?

A. Cystoscopy

B. Questionnaires and symptom scales

C. Urinalysis

D. Urinary diary

E. Urodynamics

TOG Article

Jha S, Parson M, Toozs-Hobson P. Painful bladder syndrome and interstitial cystitis. The Obstetrician and Gynaecologist 2007; 9: 34–41.

It is estimated that about 1 % of women with interstitial cystitis would eventually be diagnosed as having transitional cell carcinoma of the bladder. Therefore, some advocate that a cystoscopy is mandatory. A bladder diary would show low volumes and increased frequency but this is not diagnostic. Likewise, urodynamics would show a hypersensitive bladder with low capacity. Questionnaires (e.g., Pelvic pain and urgency/frequency scales) can be used for diagnosis but not to rule out any sinister pathology.

395 A 64-year-old patient presents with a history of increased urinary frequency, nocturia, urgency and occasional urgency incontinence.

What would be the next line of management?

A. Cystoscopy
B. Trial of anticholinergic medication
C. **Urinalysis**
D. Urinary diary
E. Urodynamics

TOG Article

Saleh S, Majumdar A, Williams K. The conservative (non-pharmacological) management of female urinary incontinence .The Obstetrician & Gynaecologist 2014; 16:169–77.

The first investigation for a patient with urinary symptoms should be a urinalysis followed by a urinary diary.

396 An 84-year-old patient presents with symptoms of urgency, urgency incontinence and nocturia. The patient is taking several different medications for other medical conditions. A diagnosis of overactive bladder is made.

The general practitioner has already tried Oxybutynin but the patient had side effects (central nervous system) and this was stopped.

Which anticholinergic medication would you now consider?

A. Darifenacin
B. Fesotrodine
C. Solifenacin
D. Tolterodine
E. **Trospium chloride**

TOG Article

Munjuluri N, Wong W, Yoong W. Anticholinergic drugs for overactive bladder: a review of the literature and practical guide. The Obstetrician and Gynaecologist 2007; 9; 9–14.

Trospium chloride has a low incidence of side effects on the central nervous system as it does not cross the blood–brain barrier. It also has less drug interaction and therefore is suitable in elderly patients who are on multiple medications.

397 A 52-year-old patient presents with a history suggestive of an overactive bladder, but also complains of fecal incontinence.

The patient has tried conservative measures and various anticholinergics with no significant benefit.

Urodynamic testing confirms detrusor overactivity and some voiding dysfunction.

M18 UROGYNAECOLOGY & PELVIC FLOOR PROBLEMS

What is the best surgical option for this patient?

A. Augmentation cystoplasty

B. Botulinum toxin injections to the bladder and teaching the patient intermittent self-catheterisation

C. Intravesical therapy (Oxybutynin)

D. Posterior tibial nerve stimulation

E. Sacral neuromodulation

TOG Article

Abboudi, H., Fynes, M. M. and Doumouchtsis, S. K. (2011), Contemporary therapy for the overactive bladder. The Obstetrician & Gynaecologist, 13: 98–106.

Sacral neuromodulation is employed to treat patients with an overactive bladder and who have not responded to medication therapy. It is also successful in treating patients with fecal incontinence and voiding dysfunction. All other treatments may help only with the overactive bladder symptoms.

398 You have just completed a vaginal hysterectomy for a procedentia. However, upon catheterisation, no urine is present in the catheter bag.

A cystoscopy is performed and no bladder trauma is identified. In order to assess ureteric function you give indigo carmine and after 5 minutes you observe a blue stream from the right ureteric orifice but none from the left.

What would be the next line of management?

A. Contact the urologist with a view to stenting the ureter

B. Cut the sutures that you used for vault support and see if there is any change in your cystoscopy findings

C. Give an intravenous a bolus dose of a diuretic and wait another 5–10 minutes

D. Insert a catheter into the bladder and perform postoperative imaging

E. Perform an intra operative ultrasound

TOG Article

Minas V, Gul N, Aust T, Doyle M, Rowlands D. Urinary tract injuries in laparoscopic gynaecological surgery; prevention, recognition and management. The Obstetrician & Gynaecologist 2014; 16:19–28.

The jet of indigo carmine can take over 5 minutes to become apparent. In the interim, one can give a diuretic and also reconfirm from the documented history to ensure there is nothing of significance in the past history (e.g., a past history of a nephrectomy).

399 A 48-year-old morbidly obese woman has a sister who recently had surgical treatment for prolapse.

She is therefore interested in finding more about the impact of obesity on the development of prolapse.

The occurrence of which type of prolapse shows the most significant increase in association with morbid obesity?

A. Cystocele

B. Enterocele

C. Rectocele

D. Urethral prolapse

E. Uterine prolapse

TOG Article

Jain, P. and Parsons, M. (2011), The effects of obesity on the pelvic floor. The Obstetrician & Gynaecologist, 13:133–142.

Hendrix et al reported that morbid obesity was associated with a significant increase in the occurrence of uterine prolapse (40%), rectocoele (75%) and cystocele (57%).

400 A woman is contemplating having either a Sacrospinouscolpopexy (no mesh) or a Sacrocolpopexy (with mesh).

The patient is keen on having a Sacrocolpopexy but is concerned about novo prolapse.

What is the incidence of de novo prolapse (cystocele), after Sacrocolpopexy and Sacrospinouscolpopexy?

	Sacrocolpopexy	Sacrospinouscolpopexy
A.	2%	4%
B.	8%	8%
C.	14%	12%
D.	24%	12%
E.	**31%**	**14%**

NICE IPG283 Sacrocolpopexy Using Mesh for Vaginal Vault Prolapse Repair

A randomized controlled trial that compared Sacrocolpopexy (mesh) with Sacrospinouscolpopexy (no mesh) reported mesh erosion after Sacrocolpopexy in 2%. De novo prolapse (cystocele) occurred in 31% (10/32) of women in the Sacrocolpopexy group and 14% (4/28) of women in the Sacrospinouscolpopexy group.